World Health Organization Classification of Tumours

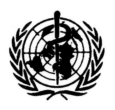

WHO   OMS

International Agency for Research on Cancer (IARC)

Pathology and Genetics of Tumours of the Digestive System

Edited by

Stanley R. Hamilton
Lauri A. Aaltonen

IARCPress
Lyon, 2000

World Health Organization Classification of Tumours

Series Editors   Paul Kleihues, M.D.
Leslie H. Sobin, M.D.

Pathology and Genetics of Tumours of the Digestive System

Editors   Stanley R. Hamilton, M.D.
Lauri A. Aaltonen, M.D., Ph.D.

Clinical Editor   René Lambert, M.D

Editorial Assistance   Wojciech Biernat, M.D.
Norman J. Carr, M.D.
Anna Sankila, M.D.

Layout   Sibylle Söring
Felix Krönert

Illustrations   Georges Mollon
Sibylle Söring

Printed by   Team Rush
69603 Villeurbanne, France

Publisher   IARCPress
International Agency for
Research on Cancer (IARC)
69372 Lyon, France

This volume was produced in collaboration with the

International Academy of Pathology (IAP)

and
with support from the

Swiss Federal Office of Public Health, Bern

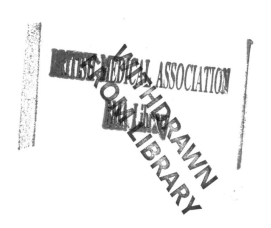

The WHO Classification of Tumours of the Digestive System
presented in this book reflects the views of a
Working Group that convened for an
Editorial and Consensus Conference in
Lyon, France, November 6-9, 1999.

Members of the Working Group are indicated
in the List of Contributors on page 253.

Published by IARC Press, International Agency for Research on Cancer,
150 cours Albert Thomas, F-69372 Lyon, France

Format for bibliographic citations:
Hamilton S.R., Aaltonen L.A. (Eds.): World Health Organization Classification of
Tumours. Pathology and Genetics of Tumours of the Digestive System. IARC Press:
Lyon 2000

IARC Library Cataloguing in Publication Data
Pathology and genetics of tumours of the digestive system / editors, S.R. Hamilton
and L.A. Aaltonen

(World Health Classification of tumours ; 2)

1. Digestive System Neoplasms I. Aaltonen, L.A. II. Hamilton, S.R.
III. Series

ISBN 92 832 2410 8   (NLM Classification: W1)

Contents

Diagnostic terms and definitions[1]

Intraepithelial neoplasia[2]. A lesion characterized by morphological changes that include altered architecture and abnormalities in cytology and differentiation. It results from clonal alterations in genes and carries a predisposition for progression to invasion and metastasis.

High-grade intraepithelial neoplasia. A mucosal change with cytologic and architectural features of malignancy but without evidence of invasion into the stroma. It includes lesions termed severe dysplasia and carcinoma in situ.

Polyp. A generic term for any excrescence or growth protruding above a mucous membrane. Polyps can be pedunculated or sessile, and are readily seen by macroscopic examination or conventional endoscopy.

Adenoma. A circumscribed benign lesion composed of tubular and/or villous structures showing intraepithelial neoplasia. The neoplastic epithelial cells are immature and typically have enlarged, hyperbasophilic and stratified nuclei.

Tubular adenoma. An adenoma in which branching tubules surrounded by lamina propria comprise at least 80% of the tumour.

Villous adenoma. An adenoma in which leaf-like or finger-like processes of lamina propria covered by dysplastic epithelium comprise at least 80% of the tumour.

Tubulovillous adenoma. An adenoma composed of both tubular and villous structures, each comprising more than 20% of the tumour.

Serrated adenoma. An adenoma composed of saw-toothed glands.

Intraepithelial neoplasia (dysplasia) associated with chronic inflammatory diseases. A neoplastic glandular epithelial proliferation occurring in a patient with a chronic inflammatory bowel disease, but with macroscopic and microscopic features that distinguish it from an adenoma, e.g. patchy distribution of dysplasia and poor circumscription.

Peutz-Jeghers polyp. A hamartomatous polyp composed of branching bands of smooth muscle covered by normal-appearing or hyperplastic glandular mucosa indigenous to the site.

Juvenile polyp. A hamartomatous polyp with a spherical head composed of tubules and cysts, lined by normal epithelium, embedded in an excess of lamina propria. In juvenile polyposis, the polyps are often multilobated with a papillary configuration and a higher ratio of glands to lamina propria.

Adenocarcinoma. A malignant epithelial tumour with glandular differentiation.

Mucinous adenocarcinoma. An adenocarcinoma containing extracellular mucin comprising more than 50% of the tumour. Note that 'mucin producing' is not synonymous with mucinous in this context.

Signet-ring cell carcinoma. An adenocarcinoma in which the predominant component (more than 50%) is composed of isolated malignant cells containing intracytoplasmic mucin.

Squamous cell (epidermoid) carcinoma. A malignant epithelial tumour with squamous cell differentiation.

Adenosquamous carcinoma. A malignant epithelial tumour with significant components of both glandular and squamous differentiation.

Small cell carcinoma. A malignant epithelial tumour similar in morphology, immunophenotype and behaviour to small cell carcinoma of the lung.

Medullary carcinoma. A malignant epithelial tumour in which the cells form solid sheets and have abundant eosinophilic cytoplasm and large, vesicular nuclei with prominent nucleoli. An intraepithelial infiltrate of lymphocytes is characteristic.

Undifferentiated carcinoma. A malignant epithelial tumour with no glandular structures or other features to indicate definite differentiation.

Carcinoid. A well differentiated neoplasm of the diffuse endocrine system.

---

[1] This list of terms is proposed to be used for the entire digestive system and reflects the view of the Working Group convened in Lyon, 6 – 9 November, 1999. Terminology evolves with scientific progress; the terms listed here reflect current understanding of the process of malignant transformation in the digestive tract. The Working Group anticipates a further convergence of diagnostic terms throughout the digestive system.

[2] In an attempt to resolve confusion surrounding the terms 'dysplasia', 'carcinoma in situ,' and 'atypia', the Working Group adopted the term 'intraepithelial neoplasia' to indicate preinvasive neoplastic change of the epithelium. The diagnosis does not exclude the possibility of coexisting carcinoma. Intraepithelial neoplasia should *not* be used as a generic description of epithelial abnormalities due to reactive or regenerative changes.

CHAPTER 1

Tumours of the Oesophagus

Carcinomas of the oesophagus pose a considerable medical and public health challenge in many parts of the world. Morphologically and aetiologically, two major types are distinguished:

Squamous cell carcinoma
In Western countries, oesophageal carcinomas with squamous cell differentiation typically arise after many years of tobacco and alcohol abuse. They frequently carry G:C >T:A mutations of the *TP53* gene. Other causes include chronic mucosal injury through hot beverages and malnutrition, but the very high incidence rates observed in Iran and some African and Asian regions remain inexplicable.

Adenocarcinoma
Oesophageal carcinomas with glandular differentiation are typically located in the distal oesophagus and occur predominantly in white males of industrialized countries, with a marked tendency for increasing incidence rates. The most important aetiological factor is chronic gastro-oesophageal reflux leading to Barrett type mucosal metaplasia, the most common precursor lesion of adenocarcinoma.

WHO histological classification of oesophageal tumours

Epithelial tumours

Squamous cell papilloma   8052/0[1]

Intraepithelial neoplasia[2]
- Squamous
- Glandular (adenoma)

Carcinoma

Squamous cell carcinoma	8070/3
Verrucous (squamous) carcinoma	8051/3
Basaloid squamous cell carcinoma	8083/3
Spindle cell (squamous) carcinoma	8074/3
Adenocarcinoma	8140/3
Adenosquamous carcinoma	8560/3
Mucoepidermoid carcinoma	8430/3
Adenoid cystic carcinoma	8200/3
Small cell carcinoma	8041/3
Undifferentiated carcinoma	8020/3
Others	

Carcinoid tumour   8240/3

Non-epithelial tumours

Leiomyoma	8890/0
Lipoma	8850/0
Granular cell tumour	9580/0
Gastrointestinal stromal tumour	8936/1
benign	8936/0
uncertain malignant potential	8936/1
malignant	8936/3
Leiomyosarcoma	8890/3
Rhabdomyosarcoma	8900/3
Kaposi sarcoma	9140/3
Malignant melanoma	8720/3
Others	

Secondary tumours

---

[1] Morphology code of the International Classification of Diseases for Oncology (ICD-O) {542} and the Systematized Nomenclature of Medicine (http://snomed.org). Behaviour is coded /0 for benign tumours, /1 for unspecified, borderline or uncertain behaviour, /2 for in situ carcinomas and grade III intraepithelial neoplasia, and /3 for malignant tumours.

[2] Intraepithelial neoplasia does not have a generic code in ICD-O. ICD-O codes are available only for lesions categorized as glandular intraepithelial neoplasia grade III (8148/2), squamous intraepithelial neoplasia, grade III (8077/2), and squamous cell carcinoma in situ (8070/2).

TNM classification of oesophageal tumours

TNM classification[1]

T – Primary Tumour

TX	Primary tumour cannot be assessed
T0	No evidence of primary tumour
Tis	Carcinoma in situ
T1	Tumour invades lamina propria or submucosa
T2	Tumour invades muscularis propria
T3	Tumour invades adventitia
T4	Tumour invades adjacent structures

N – Regional Lymph Nodes

NX	Regional lymph nodes cannot be assessed
N0	No regional lymph node metastasis
N1	Regional lymph node metastasis

M – Distant Metastasis

MX	Distant metastasis cannot be assessed
M0	No distant metastasis
M1	Distant metastasis

For tumours of lower thoracic oesophagus

	M1a	Metastasis in coeliac lymph nodes
	M1b	Other distant metastasis

For tumours of upper thoracic oesophagus

	M1a	Metastasis in cervical lymph nodes
	M1b	Other distant metastasis

For tumours of mid-thoracic oesophagus

	M1a	Not applicable
	M1b	Non-regional lymph node or other distant metastasis

Stage Grouping

Stage 0	Tis	N0	M0
Stage I	T1	N0	M0
Stage IIA	T2	N0	M0
	T3	N0	M0
Stage IIB	T1	N1	M0
	T2	N1	M0
Stage III	T3	N1	M0
	T4	Any N	M0
Stage IVA	Any T	Any N	M1a
Stage IVB	Any T	Any N	M1b

---

[1] {1, 66}. This classification applies only to carcinomas.

[2] A help desk for specific questions about the TNM classification is available at http://tnm.uicc.org.

Squamous cell carcinoma of the oesophagus

H.E. Gabbert
T. Shimoda
P. Hainaut

Y. Nakamura
J.K. Field
H. Inoue

Definition

Squamous cell carcinoma (SCC) of the oesophagus is a malignant epithelial tumour with squamous cell differentiation, microscopically characterised by keratinocyte-like cells with intercellular bridges and/or keratinization.

ICD-O Code 8070/3

Epidemiology

Squamous cell carcinoma of the oesophagus shows great geographical diversity in incidence, mortality and sex ratio. In Western countries, the age-standardized annual incidence in most areas does not exceed 5 per 100,000 population in males and 1 in females. There are, however, several well-defined high-risk areas, e.g. Normandy and Calvados in North-West France, and Northern Italy, where incidence may be as high as 30 per 100,000 population in males and 2 in females {1020, 1331}. This type of cancer is much more frequent in Eastern countries and in many developing countries. Regions with very high incidence rates have been identified in Iran, Central China, South Africa and Southern Brazil. In the city of Zhengzhou, capital of Henan province in China, the mortality rate exceeds 100 per 100,000 population in males and 50 in females {1116, 2191}.

In both high-risk and low-risk regions, this cancer is exceedingly rare before the age of 30 and the median age is around 65 in both males and females. Recent changes in the distribution pattern in France indicate that the rate of SCC has increased steadily in low-risk areas, particularly among females, whereas there may be a slight decrease in high-risk areas. In the United States, a search in hospitalisation records of military veterans indicates that SCC is 2-3 times more frequent among blacks than among Asians, Whites or Native Americans {453}.

Aetiology

Tobacco and alcohol. In Western countries, nearly 90% of the risk of SCC can be attributed to tobacco and alcohol. Each of these factors influences the risk of oesophageal cancer in a different way. With regard to the consumption of tobacco, a moderate intake during a long period carries a higher risk than a high intake during a shorter period, whereas the reverse is true for alcohol. Both factors combined show a multiplicative effect, even at low alcohol intake. In high-risk areas of North-West France and Northern Italy, local drinking customs may partially explain the excess incidence of SCC {523, 1020}. In Japanese alcoholics, a

polymorphism in *ALDH2*, the gene encoding aldehyde dehydrogenase 2, has been shown to be significantly associated with several cancers of the upper digestive tract, including squamous cell cancer. This observation suggests a role for acetaldehyde, one of the main carcinogenic metabolites of alcohol in the development of oesophageal carcinoma {2177}.

Nutrition. Risk factors other than tobacco and alcohol play significant roles in other regions of the world. In high-risk areas of China, a deficiency in certain trace elements and the consumption of pickled or mouldy foods (which are potential sources of nitrosamines) have been suggested.

Hot beverages. Worldwide, one of the most common risk factors appears to be the consumption of burning-hot beverages (such as Mate tea in South America) which cause thermal injury leading to chronic oesophagitis and then to precancerous lesions {1116, 2191, 387}.

HPV. Conflicting reports have proposed a role for infectious agents, including human papillomavirus (HPV) infection. Although HPV DNA is consistently detected in 20 to 40% of SCC in high-risk areas of China, it is generally absent in the cancers arising in Western countries {954, 679}.

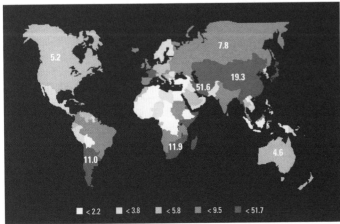

Fig. 1.01 Worldwide annual incidence (per 100,000) of oesophageal cancer in males. Numbers on the map indicate regional average values.

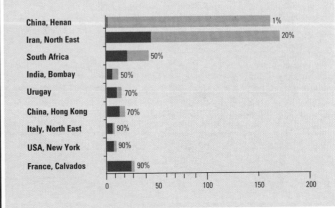

Fig. 1.02 Squamous cell carcinoma of the oesophagus. Age-standardized incidence rates per 100,000 and proportions (%) due to alcohol and tobacco (dark-blue).

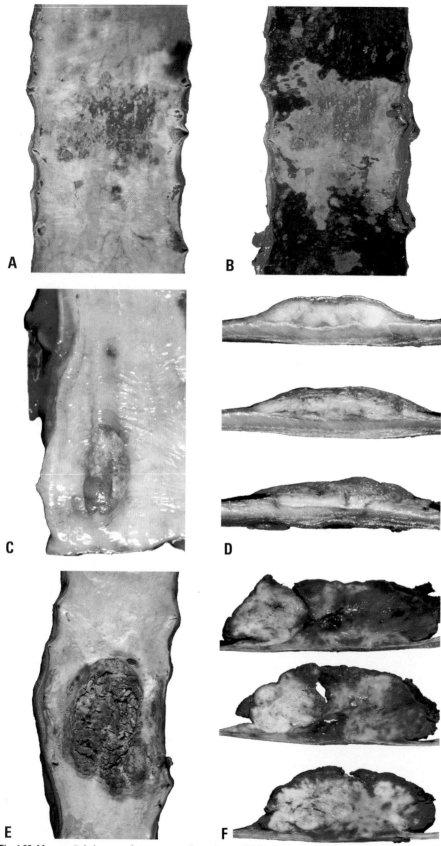

Associations between achalasia, Plummer-Vinson syndrome, coeliac disease and tylosis (focal nonepidermolytic palmoplantar keratoderma) with oesophageal cancer have also been described.

Localization
Oesophageal SCC is located predominantly in the middle and the lower third of the oesophagus, only 10-15% being situated in the upper third {1055}.

Clinical features
Symptoms and signs
The most common symptoms of advanced oesophageal cancer are dysphagia, weight loss, retrosternal or epigastric pain, and regurgitation caused by narrowing of the oesophageal lumen by tumour growth {606}. Superficial SCC usually has no specific symptoms but sometimes causes a tingling sensation, and is, therefore, often detected incidentally during upper gastrointestinal endoscopy {464, 1874}.

Endoscopy and vital staining
Superficial oesophageal cancer is commonly observed as a slight elevation or shallow depression on the mucosal surface, which is a minor morphological change compared to that of advanced cancer. Macroscopically, three types can be distinguished: flat, polypoid and ulcerated. Chromoendoscopy utilizing toluidine blue or Lugol iodine spray may be of value {465, 481}. Toluidine blue, a metachromatic stain from the thiazine group, has a particular affinity for RNA and DNA, and stains areas that are richer in nuclei than the normal mucosa. Lugol solution reacts specifically with glycogen in the normal squamous epithelium, whereas precancerous and cancerous lesions, but also inflamed areas and gastric heterotopia, are not stained. However, the superficial extension of carcinomas confined to the mucosa can not be clearly recognized by simple endoscopy.

Endoscopic ultrasonography
Endoscopic ultrasonography is used to evaluate both depth of tumour infiltration and para-oesophageal lymph node involvement in early and advanced stages of the disease {1509, 1935}. For the evaluation of the depth of infiltration, high frequency endoscopic ultrasonography may be used {1302}. In general,

Fig. 1.03 Macroscopic images of squamous cell carcinoma (SCC) of the oesophagus. **A** Flat superficial type. **B** Lugol iodine staining of the specimen illustrated in A. **C** Polypoid SCC. **D** Longitudinal sections of carcinoma illustrated in C. **E** Deeply invasive polypoid SCC. **F** Longitudinal sections of carcinoma illustrated in E.

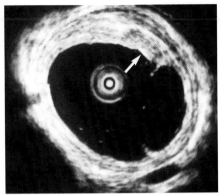

Fig. 1.04 Catheter probe ultrasonograph of a squamous cell carcinoma, presenting as hypoechoic lesion (arrow).

oesophageal carcinoma presents on endosonography as a circumscribed or diffuse wall thickening with a predominantly echo-poor or echo-inhomogeneous pattern. As a result of tumour penetration through the wall and into surrounding structures, the endosonographic wall layers are destroyed.

Computed tomography (CT) and magnetic resonance imaging (MRI)
In advanced carcinomas, CT and MRI give information on local and systemic spread of SCC. Tumour growth is characterized as swelling of the oesophageal wall, with or without direct invasion to surrounding organs {1518}. Cervical, abdominal and mediastinal node enlargement is recorded. Three-dimensional CT or MRI images may be presented as virtual endoscopy, effectively demonstrating T2-T4 lesions, but not T1 lesions.

Macroscopy
The gross appearance varies according to whether it is detected in an early or an advanced stage of the disease. Among early SCC, polypoid, plaque-like, depressed and occult lesions have been described {161, 2183}. For the macroscopic classification of advanced oesophageal SCC, Ming {1236} has proposed three major patterns: fungating, ulcerative, and infiltrating. The fungating pattern is characterized by a predominantly exophytic growth, whereas in the ulcerative pattern, the tumour growth is predominantly intramural, with a central ulceration and elevated ulcer edges. The infiltrative pattern, which is the least common one, also shows a predominantly intramural growth, but causes only a small mucosal defect. Similar types of macroscopic

growth patterns have been defined in the classification of the Japanese Society for Esophageal Diseases {58}.

Tumour spread and staging
For the staging of SCC, the TNM system (tumour, node, metastasis) established by the International Union Against Cancer (UICC) is the most widely used system. Its usefulness in the planning of treatment and in the prediction of prognosis has been validated {1104, 895, 66, 1, 772}.

Superficial oesophageal carcinoma.
When the tumour is confined to the mucosa or the submucosa, the term superficial oesophageal carcinoma is used irrespective of the presence of regional lymph node metastases {58, 161}. In China and in Japan, the term early oesophageal carcinoma is often used defining a carcinoma that invades no deeper than the submucosa but has not metastasised {609}. In several studies from Japan, superficial carcinomas accounted for 10-20% of all resected carcinomas, whereas in Western countries

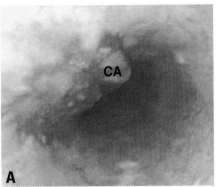

A

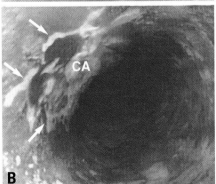

B

Fig. 1.05 A Endoscopic view of a superficial squamous cell carcinoma presenting as a large nodule (CA) in a zone of erosion. **B** After spraying of 2% iodine solution, the superficial extent of the tumour becomes visible as unstained light yellow area (CA, arrows).

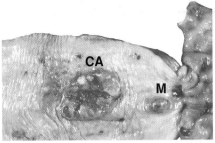

Fig. 1.06 Primary squamous cell carcinoma (CA) of oesophagus with an intramural metastasis (M) near the oesophagogastric junction.

superficial carcinomas are much less frequently reported {543}. About 5% of superficial carcinomas that have invaded the lamina propria display lymph node metastases, whereas in carcinomas that invade the submucosa the risk of nodal metastasis is about 35% {1055}. For tumours that have infiltrated beyond the submucosa, the term advanced oesophageal carcinoma is applied.

Intramural metastases. A special feature of oesophageal SCC is the occurrence of intramural metastases, which have been found in resected oesophageal specimens in 11-16% of cases {896, 987}. These metastases are thought to result from intramural lymphatic spread with the establishment of secondary intramural tumour deposits. Intramural metastases are associated with an advanced stage of disease and with shorter survival.

Second primary SCC. Additionally, the occurrence of multiple independent SCC has been described in between 14 and 31% of cases, the second cancers being mainly carcinomas *in situ* and superficial SCC {1154, 989, 1507}.

Treatment groups. Following the clinical staging, patients are usually divided into two treatment groups: those with locoregional disease in whom the tumour is potentially curable (e.g. by surgery, radiotherapy, multimodal therapy), and those with advanced disease (metastases outside the regional area or invasion of the airway) in whom only palliative treatment is indicated {606}. Oesophageal SCC limited to the mucosa may be treated by endoscopic mucosal resection due to its low risk of nodal metastasis. Endoscopic mucosal resection is also indicated for high-grade intraepithelial neoplasia. Tumours that have invaded the submucosa or those in more advanced tumour stages have more than 30% risk of lymph node metastasis, and endoscopic therapy is not indicated {465}. Additionally, clinical staging is performed in order to determine the success of treatment, e.g. following radio- and/or chemotherapy.

Tumour spread

The most common sites of metastasis of oesophageal SCC are the regional lymph nodes. The risk of lymph node metastasis is about 5% in carcinomas confined to the mucosa but over 30% in carcinomas invading the submucosa and over 80% in carcinomas invading adjacent organs or tissues {772}. Lesions of the upper third of the oesophagus most frequently involve cervical and mediastinal lymph nodes, whereas those of the middle third metastasise to the mediastinal, cervical and upper gastric lymph nodes. Carcinomas of the lower third preferentially spread to the lower mediastinal and the abdominal lymph nodes {28}. The most common sites of haematogenous metastases are the lung and the liver {1153, 1789}. Less frequently affected sites are the bones, adrenal glands, and brain {1551}. Recently, disseminated tumour cells were identified by means of immunostaining in the bone marrow of about 40% of patients with oesophageal SCC {1933}. Recurrence of cancer following oesophageal resection can be locoregional or distant, both with approximately equal frequency {1185, 1027}.

Histopathology

Oesophageal SCC is defined as the penetration of neoplastic squamous epithelium through the epithelial basement membrane and extension into the lamina propria or deeper tissue layers. Invasion commonly starts from a carcinoma in situ with the proliferation of rete-like projections of neoplastic epithelium that push into the lamina propria with subsequent dissociation into small carcinomatous cell clusters. Along with vertical tumour cell infiltration, usually a horizontal growth undermines the adjacent normal mucosa at the tumour periphery. The carcinoma may already invade intramural lymphatic vessels and veins at an early stage of disease. The frequency of lymphatic and blood vessel invasion increases with increasing depth of invasion {1662}. Tumour cells in lymphatic vessels and in blood vessels may be found progressively several centimetres beyond the gross

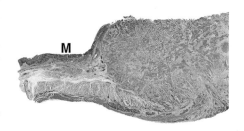

Fig. **1.07** Squamous cell carcinoma with transmural invasion. M, remaining intact mucosa.

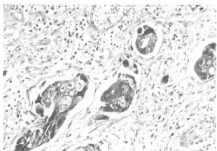

Fig. **1.08** Squamous cell carcinoma invading thin-walled lymphatic vessels.

tumour. The carcinoma invades the muscular layers, enters the loose fibrous adventitia and may extend beyond the adventitia, with invasion of adjacent organs or tissues, especially the trachea and bronchi, eventually with the formation of oesophagotracheal or oesophagobronchial fistulae {1789}.

Oesophageal SCC displays different microscopic patterns of invasion, which are categorised as 'expansive growth' or 'infiltrative growth'. The former pattern is characterized by a broad and smooth invasion front with little or no tumour cell dissociation, whereas the infiltrative pattern shows an irregular invasion front and a marked tumour cell dissociation.

The degree of desmoplastic or inflammatory stromal reaction, nuclear polymorphism and keratinization is extremely variable. Additionally, otherwise typical oesophageal SCC may contain small foci of glandular differentiation, indicated by the formation of tubular glands or mucin-producing tumour cells {987}.

Verrucous carcinoma (ICD-O 8051/3)

This rare variant of squamous cell carcinoma {19} is histologically comparable to verrucous carcinomas arising at other sites {969}. On gross examination, its appearance is exophytic, warty, cauliflower-like or papillary. It can be found in any part of the oesophagus. Histologically, it is defined as a malignant papillary tumour composed of well differentiated and keratinized squamous epithelium with minimal cytological atypia, and pushing rather than infiltrating margins {2066}. Oesophageal verrucous carcinoma grows slowly and invades locally, with a very low metastasising potential.

Spindle cell carcinoma (ICD-O 8094/3)

This unusual malignancy is defined as a squamous cell carcinoma with a variable

sarcomatoid spindle cell component. It is also known by a variety of other terms, including carcinosarcoma, pseudosarcomatous squamous cell carcinoma, polypoid carcinoma, and squamous cell carcinoma with a spindle cell component {1055}. Macroscopically, the tumour is characterized by a polypoid growth pattern. The spindle cells may be capable of maturation, forming bone, cartilage and skeletal muscle cells {662}. Alternatively, they may be more pleomorphic, resembling malignant fibrous histiocytoma. In the majority of cases a gradual transition between carcinomatous and sarcomatous components has been observed on the light microscopic level. Immunohistochemical and electron microscopic studies indicate that the sarcomatous spindle cells show various degrees of epithelial differentiation. Therefore, the sarcoma-

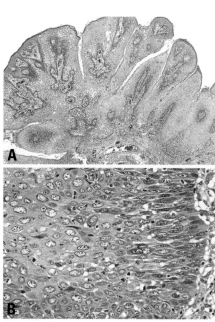

Fig. **1.09** Verrucous carcinoma. **A** Typical exophytic papillary growth. **B** High degree of differentiation.

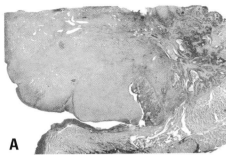
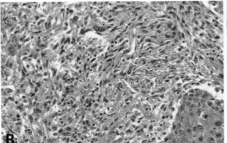
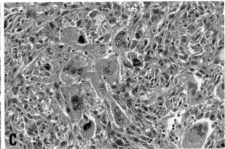

Fig. 1.10 Spindle cell carcinoma. **A** Typical polypoid appearance. **B** Transition between conventional and spindle cells areas. **C** Malignant fibrous histiocytoma-like area in a spindle cell carcinoma.

tous component may be metaplastic. However, a recent molecular analysis of a single case of a spindle cell carcinoma showed divergent genetic alterations in the carcinomatous and in the sarcomatous tumour component suggesting two independent malignant cell clones {823}.

Basaloid squamous cell carcinoma (ICD-O 8083/3)

This rare but distinct variant of oesophageal SCC {1961} appears to be identical to the basaloid squamous cell carcinomas of the upper aerodigestive tract {109}. Histologically, it is composed of closely packed cells with hyperchromatic nuclei and scant basophilic cytoplasm, which show a solid growth pattern, small gland-like spaces and foci of comedo-type necrosis. Basaloid squamous cell carcinomas are associated

with intraepithelial neoplasia, invasive SCC, or islands of squamous differentiation among the basaloid cells {2036}. The proliferative activity is higher than in typical SCC. However, basaloid squamous cell carcinoma is also characterized by a high rate of apoptosis and its prognosis does not differ significantly from that of the ordinary oesophageal SCC {1663}.

Precursor lesions

Most studies on precursor lesions of oesophageal SCC have been carried out in high-risk populations, especially in Iran and Northern China, but there is no evidence that precursor lesions in low-risk regions are substantially different. The development of oesophageal SCC is thought to be a multistage process which progresses from the conversion of normal squamous epithelium to that with basal cell hyperplasia, intraepithelial neoplasia (dysplasia and carcinoma in situ), and, finally, invasive SCC {354, 1547, 377}.

Intraepithelial neoplasia. This lesion is about eight times more common in high cancer-risk areas than in low-risk areas {1547}, and is frequently found adjacent to invasive SCC in oesophagectomy specimens {1154, 988}. Morphological features of intraepithelial neoplasia include both architectural and cytological abnormalities. The architectural abnormality is characterized by a disorganisation of the epithelium and loss of normal cell polarity. Cytologically, the cells exhibit irregular and hyperchromatic nuclei, an increase in nuclear/cytoplasmic ratio and increased mitotic activity. Dysplasia is usually graded as low or high-grade. In low-grade dysplasia, the abnormalities are often confined to the lower half of the epithelium, whereas in high-grade dysplasia the abnormal cells also occur in

the upper half and exhibit a greater degree of atypia. In carcinoma *in situ*, the atypical cells are present throughout the epithelium without evidence of maturation at the surface of the epithelium {1154}. In a two-tier system, severe dysplasia and carcinoma-in-situ are included under the rubric of high-grade intraepithelial neoplasia, and may have the same clinical implications {1055}.

Epidemiological follow-up studies suggest an increased risk for the subsequent development of invasive SCC for patients with basal cell hyperplasia (relative risk: 2.1), low-grade dysplasia (RR: 2.2), moderate-grade dysplasia (RR: 15.8), high-grade dysplasia (RR: 72.6) and carcinoma in situ (RR: 62.5) {377}.

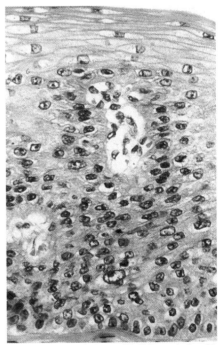

Fig. 1.11 Basaloid squamous cell carcinoma. **A** Typical comedo-type necrosis. **B** Small gland-like structures.

Fig. 1.12 Low-grade intraepithelial neoplasia with an increase in basal cells, loss of polarity in the deep epithelium and slight cytological atypia.

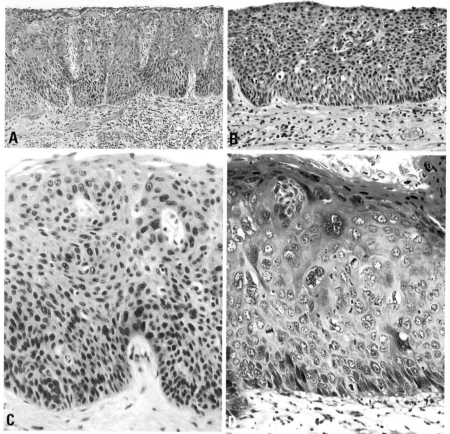

Fig. 1.13 High grade intraepithelial neoplasia of oesophageal squamous epithelium. Architectural disarray, loss of polarity and cellular atypia are much greater than shown in Fig. 1.12. Changes in **D** extend to the parakeratotic layer of the luminal surface.

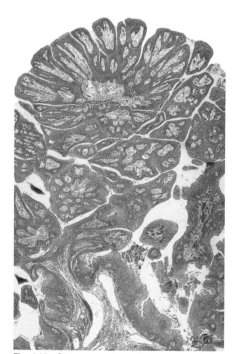

Fig. 1.14 Squamous cell papilloma of distal oesophagus. This lesion was negative for human papillomavirus by in situ hybridisation.

Basal cell hyperplasia
This lesion is histologically defined as an otherwise normal squamous epithelium with a basal zone thickness greater than 15% of total epithelial thickness, without elongation of lamina propria papillae {377}. In most cases, basal cell hyperplasia is an epithelial proliferative lesion in response to oesophagitis, which is frequently observed in high-risk populations for oesophageal cancer {1547}.

Squamous cell papilloma (ICD-O 8052/0)
Squamous cell papilloma is rare and usually causes no specific symptoms. It is a benign tumour composed of hyperplastic squamous epithelium covering finger-like processes with cores derived from the lamina propria. The polypoid lesions are smooth, sharply demarcated, and usually 5 mm or less in maximum diameter {249, 1428}. Rarely, giant papillomas have been reported, with sizes up to 5 cm {2037}. Most squamous cell papillomas represent single isolated lesions, typically located in the distal to

middle third of the oesophagus, but multiple lesions occur.
Histologically, cores of fibrovascular tissue are covered by mature stratified squamous epithelium. The aetiological role of human papillomavirus (HPV) infection has been investigated in several studies, but the results were inconclusive {248}. Malignant progression to SCC is extremely rare.
In Japan, oesophageal squamous cell carcinoma is diagnosed mainly based on nuclear criteria, even in cases judged to be non-invasive intraepithelial neoplasia (dysplasia) in the West. This difference in diagnostic practice may contribute to the relatively high rate of incidence and good prognosis of superficial squamous cell carcinoma reported in Japan {1682}.

Grading
Grading of oesophageal SCC is traditionally based on the parameters of mitotic activity, anisonucleosis and degree of differentiation.
Well differentiated tumours have cytological and histological features similar to those of the normal oesophageal squamous epithelium. In well differentiated oesophageal SCC there is a high proportion of large, differentiated, keratinocyte-like squamous cells and a low proportion of small basal-type cells, which are located in the periphery of the cancer cell nests {1055}. The occurrence of keratinization has been interpreted as a sign of differentiation, although the normal oesophageal squamous epithelium does not keratinize.
Poorly differentiated tumours predominantly consist of basal-type cells, which usually exhibit a high mitotic rate.
Moderately differentiated carcinomas, between the well and poorly differentiated types, are the most common type, accounting for about two-thirds of all oesophageal SCC. However, since no generally accepted criteria have been identified to score the relative contribution of the different grading parameters, grading of SCC suffers from a great interobserver variation.
Undifferentiated carcinomas are defined by a lack of definite light microscopic features of differentiation. However, ultrastructural or immunohistochemical investigations may disclose features of squamous differentiation in a subset of light-microscopically undifferentiated carcinomas {1881}.

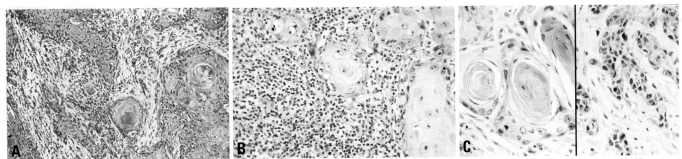

Fig. 1.15 Squamous cell carcinoma. **A** Moderately differentiated. **B** Well differentiated with prominent lymphoid infiltrate. **C** Well differentiated areas (left) contrast with immature basal-type cells of a poorly differentiated carcinoma (right).

Genetic susceptibility

Familial predisposition of oesophageal cancer has been only poorly studied except in its association with focal non-epidermolytic palmoplantar keratoderma (NEPPK or tylosis) {1279, 1278, 752}. This autosomal, dominantly inherited disorder of the palmar and plantar surfaces of the skin segregates together with oesophageal cancer in three pedigrees, two of which are extensive {456, 1834, 693}. The causative locus has been designated the tylosis oesophageal cancer (TOC) gene and maps to 17q25 between the anonymous microsatellite markers D17S1839 and D17S785 {1594, 899}. The genetic defect is thought to be in a molecule involved in the physical structure of stratified squamous epithelia whereby loss of function of the gene may alter oesophageal integrity thereby making it more susceptible to environmental mutagens.

Several structural candidate genes such as envoplakin (EVPL), integrin β4 (ITGB4) and plakoglobin have been excluded as the TOC gene following integration of the genetic and physical maps of this region {1595}. The importance of this gene in a larger population than those afflicted with the familial disease is indicated by the association of the genomic region containing the TOC gene with sporadic squamous cell oesophageal carcinomas {2020, 823}, Barrett adenocarcinoma of the oesophagus {439}, and primary breast cancers {549} using loss of heterozygosity studies.

Genetics

Alterations in genes that encode regulators of the G1 to S transition of cell cycle are common in SCC. Mutation in the TP53 gene (17p13) is thought to be an early event, sometimes already detectable in intraepithelial neoplasia. The frequency and type of mutation varies from one geographic area to the other, suggesting that some TP53 mutations may occur as the result of exposure to region-specific, exogenous risk factors. However, even in SCC from Western Europe, the TP53 mutation spectrum does not show the same tobacco-associated mutations as in lung cancers {1266}. Amplification of cyclin D1 (11q13) occurs in 20-40% of SCC and is frequently detected in cancers that retain expression of the Rb protein, in agreement with the notion that these two factors cooperate within the same signalling cascade {859}. Inactivation of CDKN2A occurs essentially by homozygous deletion or de novo methylation and appears to be associated with advanced cancer. Other potentially important genetic alterations include transcriptional inactivation of the FHIT gene (fragile histidine triad, a presumptive tumour suppressor on 3p14) by methylation of 5' CpG islands, and deletion of the tylosis oesophageal cancer gene on 17q25 {2020, 1264}. Furthermore, analysis of clones on 3p21.3, where frequent LOH occurs in oesophageal cancer {1274}, recently led to identification of a novel gene termed DLC1 (deleted in lung and oesophageal cancer-1) {365}. Although the function of the DLC1 gene remains to be clarified, RT-PCR experiments indicated that 33% of primary cancers of lung and oesophagus lacked DLC1 transcripts entirely or contained increased levels of nonfunctional DLC1 mRNA. Recent evidence suggests that LOH at a new, putative tumour suppressor locus on 5p15 may occur in a majority of SCC {1497}. Amplification of several proto-oncogenes has also been reported (HST-1, HST-2, EGFR, MYC) {1266}. How these various genetic events correlate with phenotypic

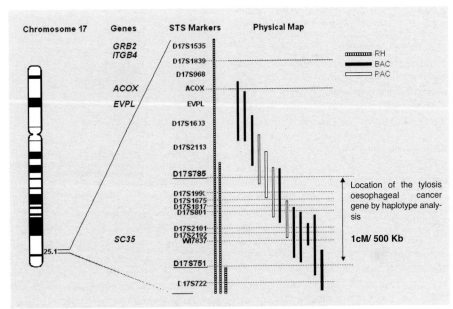

Fig. 1.16 Location of the tylosis oesophageal cancer gene on chromosome 17q.

changes and co operate in the sequence of events leading to SCC is still speculative.

Prognosis and prognostic factors

Overall, the prognosis of oesophageal SCC is poor and the 5-year survival rates in registries are around 10%. Cure is foreseen only for superficial cancer. The survival varies, depending upon tumour stage at diagnosis, treatment received, patient's general health status, morphological features and molecular features of the tumour. In the past, studies on prognostic factors were largely focused on patients who were treated by surgery, whereas factors influencing survival of patients treated by radiotherapy or by multimodal therapy have been investigated only rarely.

Morphological factors
The extent of spread of the oesophageal SCC is the most important factor for prognosis, the TNM classification being the most widely used staging system.
Staging. All studies indicate that the depth of invasion and the presence of nodal or distant metastases are independent predictors of survival {1104, 895, 772}. In particular, lymph node involvement, regardless of the extent of the primary tumour, indicates a poor prognosis {1862, 912, 1873}. More recently, the prognostic significance of more sophisticated methods for the determination of tumour spread have been evaluated, including the ratio of involved to resected lymph nodes {1603}, immunohistochemically determined lymph node micrometastases {824, 1327} and micrometastases in the bone marrow {1933}. However, current data are still too limited to draw final conclusions on the prognostic value.
Differentiation. The prognostic impact of tumour differentiation is equivocal, possibly due to the poor standardisation of the grading system and to the high prognostic power of tumour stage. Although some studies have shown a significant influence of tumour grade on survival {709, 772}, the majority of studies have not {443, 1858, 1601, 1660}. Other histopathological features associated with a poor prognosis include the presence of vascular and/or lymphatic invasion {772, 1662} and an infiltrative growth pattern of the primary tumour {1660}.
Lymphocytic infiltration. Intense lympho-

cytic response to the tumour has been associated with a better prognosis {1660, 443}.
Proliferation. The cancer cell proliferation index, determined immunohistochemically by antibodies such as PCNA or Ki- 67 / MIB-1, have been studied extensively. However, the proliferation index does not appear to be an independent prognostic factor {2189, 1005, 1659, 779}.

DNA ploidy. Aneuploidy of cancer cells, as determined by flow cytometry or by image analysis, has been identified in 55% to 95% of oesophageal SCC {935}. Regarding the prognostic impact, patients with diploid tumours usually survive longer than those with aneuploid tumours. However, a prognostic impact independent of tumour stage has been shown only in two studies {422, 1195}, whereas the majority of studies have not verified this

Table 1.01
Genetic alterations in squamous cell carcinoma of the oesophagus.

Gene	Location	Tumor abnormality	Function
TP53	17p13	Point mutation, LOH	G1 arrest, apoptosis, genetic stability
p16, p15, ARF/CDKN2	9p22	Homozygous loss Promoter methylation	CDK inhibitor (cell cycle control)
Cyclin D1	11q13	Amplification	Cell cycle control
EGFR	17p13	Amplification, overexpression	Signal transduction (membrane Tyr kinase)
c-myc	8q24.1	Amplification	Transcription factor
Rb	13q14	LOH Absence of expression	Cell cycle control
TOC	17q25	LOH	Tumour suppressor
FEZ1	8p22	Transcription shutdown	Transcription factor
DLC1	3p21.3	Transcription shutdown	Growth inhibition

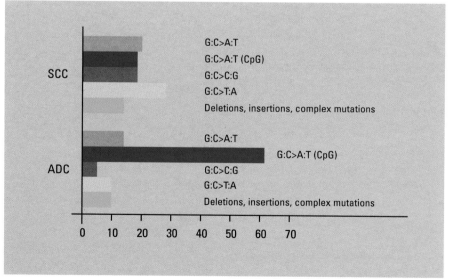

Fig. 1.17 Spectrum of *TP53* mutations in squamous cell carcinoma (SCC) and adenocarcinoma (ADC) of the oesophagus.

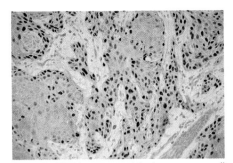

Fig. 1.18 *TP53* immunoreactivity in squamous cell carcinoma of the oesophagus.

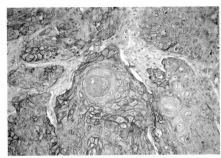

Fig. 1.19 Immunoreactivity for epidermal growth factor receptor (EGFR) in oesophageal squamous cell carcinoma.

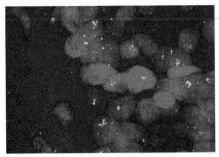

Fig. 1.20 Fluorescence in situ hybridisation demonstrating cyclin D1 in squamous carcinoma cells.

finding {935}. Therefore, the determination of DNA ploidy is currently not considered to improve the prognostic information provided by the TNM system {1055}.

Extent of resection. The frequency of locoregional recurrence is negatively correlated with the distance of the primary tumour to the proximal resection margin and possibly to preoperative chemotherapy {1890, 1027}.

Molecular factors
The *TP53* gene is mutated in 35% to 80%

of oesophageal SCC {1266}. Whereas some studies indicated a negative prognostic influence of p53 protein accumulation in cancer cell nuclei {1743, 277}, others did not observe any prognostic value of either immunoexpression or *TP53* mutation {2014, 1661, 1008, 779, 319}.

Other potential prognostic factors include growth factors and their receptors {927}, oncogenes, including *c-erbB-2* and *int-2* {778}, cell cycle regulators {1748, 1297}, tumour suppressor genes {1886}, redox

defence system components, e.g., metallothionein and heat shock proteins {897}, and matrix proteinases {1303, 1947, 2155}. Alterations of these factors in oesophageal SCC may enhance tumour cell proliferation, invasiveness, and metastatic potential, and thus may be associated with survival. However, none of the factors tested so far has entered clinical practice.

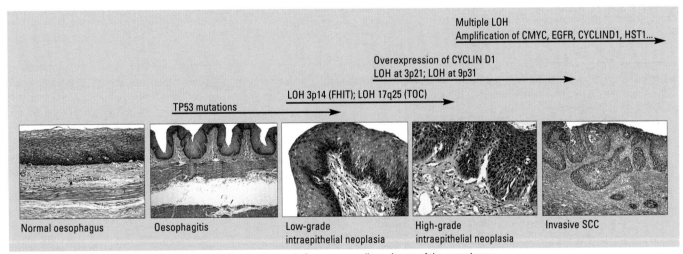

Normal oesophagus Oesophagitis Low-grade intraepithelial neoplasia High-grade intraepithelial neoplasia Invasive SCC

TP53 mutations → LOH 3p14 (FHIT); LOH 17q25 (TOC) → Overexpression of CYCLIN D1 LOH at 3p21; LOH at 9p31 → Multiple LOH Amplification of CMYC, EGFR, CYCLIND1, HST1...

Fig. 1.21 Putative sequence of genetic alterations in the development of squamous cell carcinoma of the oesophagus.

Adenocarcinoma of the oesophagus

M. Werner
J.F. Flejou
P. Hainaut
H. Höfler

R. Lambert
G. Keller
H.J. Stein

Definition

A malignant epithelial tumour of the oesophagus with glandular differentiation arising predominantly from Barrett mucosa in the lower third of the oesophagus. Infrequently, adenocarcinoma originates from heterotopic gastric mucosa in the upper oesophagus, or from mucosal and submucosal glands.

ICD-O Code   8140/3

Epidemiology

In industrialized countries, the incidence and prevalence of adenocarcinoma of the oesophagus has risen dramatically {1827}. Population based studies in the U.S.A. and several European countries indicate that the incidence of oesophageal adenocarcinoma has doubled between the early 1970s to the late 1980s and continues to increase at a rate of about 5% to 10% per year {152, 153, 370, 405, 1496}. This is paralleled by rising rates of adenocarcinoma of the gastric cardia and of subcardial gastric carcinoma. It has been estimated that the rate of increase of oesophageal and oesophagogastric junction adenocarcinoma in the U.S.A. during the past decade surpassed that of any other type of cancer {152}. In the mid 1990s the incidence of oesophageal adenocarcinoma has been estimated between 1 and 4 per 100,000 per year in the U.S.A. and several European countries and thus approaches or exceeds that of squamous cell oesophageal cancer in these regions. In Asia and Africa, adenocarcinoma of the oesophagus is an uncommon finding, but increasing rates are also reported from these areas.

In addition to the rise in incidence, adenocarcinoma of the oesophagus and of the oesophagogastric junction share some epidemiological characteristics that clearly distinguish them from squamous cell oesophageal carcinoma and adenocarcinoma of the distal stomach. These include a high preponderance for the male sex (male:female ratio 7:1), a higher incidence among whites and an average age at the time of diagnosis of around 65 years {1756}.

Aetiology

Barrett oesophagus

The epidemiological features of adenocarcinoma of the distal oesophagus and oesophagogastric junction match those of patients with known intestinal metaplasia in the distal oesophagus, i.e. Barrett oesophagus {1605, 1827}, which has been identified as the single most important precursor lesion and risk factor for adenocarcinoma of the distal oesophagus, irrespective of the length of the segment with intestinal metaplasia.

Intestinal metaplasia of the oesophagus develops when the normal squamous oesophageal epithelium is replaced by columnar epithelium during the process of healing after repetitive injury to the oesophageal mucosa, typically associated with gastro-oesophageal reflux disease {1798, 1799}.

Intestinal metaplasia can be detected in more than 80% of patients with adenocarcinoma of the distal oesophagus. {1756, 1824}. A series of prospective endoscopic surveillance studies in patients with known intestinal metaplasia of the distal oesophagus has shown an incidence of oesophageal adenocarcinoma in the order of 1/100 years of follow up {1799}. This translates into a life-time risk for oesophageal adenocarcinoma of about 10% in these patients. The length of the oesophageal segment with intestinal metaplasia, and the presence of ulcerations and strictures have been implicated as further risk factors for the development of oesophageal adenocarcinoma by some authors, but this has not been confirmed by others {1799, 1797, 1827}.

The biological significance of so-called ultrashort Barrett oesophagus or intestinal metaplasia just beneath a normal Z line has yet to be fully clarified {1325}. Whether adenocarcinoma of the gastric cardia or subcardial gastric cancer is also related to foci of intestinal metaplasia at or immediately below the gastric cardia {715, 1797, 1722} is discussed in the chapter on adenocarcinoma of the oesophagogstric junction. Despite the broad advocation of endoscopic surveillance in patients with known Barrett oesophagus, more than 50% of patients with oesophageal adenocarcinoma still have locally advanced or metastatic disease at the time of presentation {1826}.

Chronic gastro-oesophageal reflux is the usual underlying cause of the repetitive mucosal injury and also provides an abnormal environment during the healing process that predisposes to intestinal metaplasia {1799}. Data from Sweden have shown an odds ratio of 7.7 for oesophageal adenocarcinoma in persons with recurrent reflux symptoms, as compared with persons without such symptoms {1002, 1001}.

The more frequent, more severe, and longer-lasting the symptoms of reflux, the greater the risk. Among persons with long-standing and severe symptoms of reflux, the odds ratio for oesophageal adenocarcinoma was 43.5. Based on these data a strong and probably causal relation between gastro-oesophageal reflux, one of the most common benign disorders of the digestive tract, and oesophageal adenocarcinoma has been postulated.

Factors predisposing for the development of Barrett oesophagus and subsequent adenocarcinoma in patients with gastro-oesophageal reflux disease include a markedly increased oesophageal exposure time to refluxed gastric and duodenal contents due to a defective barrier function of the lower oesophageal sphincter and ineffective clearance function of the tubular oesophagus {1823, 1827}. Experimental and clinical data indicate that combined oesophageal exposure to gastric acid and duodenal contents (bile acids and pancreatic enzymes) appears to be more detrimental than isolated exposure to gastric juice or duodenal contents alone {1241, 1825}. Combined reflux is thought to increase cancer risk by promoting cellular proliferation, and by exposing the oesophageal epithelium to potentially genotoxic gastric and intestinal contents, e.g. nitrosamines {1825}.

Tobacco
Smoking has been identified as another major risk factor for oesophageal adenocarcinoma and may account for as much as 40% of cases through an early stage carcinogenic effect {562, 2204}.

Obesity
In a Swedish population-based case control study, obesity was also associated with an increased risk for oesophageal adenocarcinoma. In this study the adjusted odds ratio was 7.6 among persons in the highest body mass index (BMI) quartile compared with persons in the lowest. Obese persons (BMI > 30 kg/m²) had an odds ratio of 16.2 as compared with the leanest persons (persons with a BMI < 22 kg/m²) {1002}. The pathogenetic basis of the association with obesity remains to be elucidated {310}.

Alcohol
In contrast to squamous cell oesophageal carcinoma, there is no strong relation between alcohol consumption and adenocarcinoma of the oesophagus.

Helicobacter pylori
This infection does not appear to be a predisposing factor for the development of intestinal metaplasia and adenocarcinoma in the distal oesophagus. According to recent studies, gastric *H. pylori* infection may even exert a protective effect {309}.

Localization
Adenocarcinoma may occur anywhere in a segment lined with columnar metaplastic mucosa (Barrett oesophagus) but develops mostly in its proximal verge. Adenocarcinoma in a short segment of Barrett oesophagus is easily mistaken for adenocarcinoma of the cardia. Since adenocarcinoma originating from the distal oesophagus may infiltrate the gastric cardia and carcinoma of the gastric cardia or subcardial region may grow into the distal oesophagus these entities are frequently difficult to discriminate (see chapter on tumours of the oesophagogastric junction). As an exception, adenocarcinoma occurs also in the middle or proximal third of the oesophagus, in the

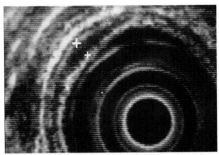

Fig. 1.22 Endoscopic ultrasonograph of Barrett T1 adenocarcinoma. The hypoechoic tumour lies between the first and second hyperechoic layers (markers). The continuity of the second layer (submucosa) is respected.

latter usually from a congenital islet of heterotopic columnar mucosa (that is present in up to 10% of the population).

Barrett oesophagus
Symptoms and signs
Barrett oesophagus as the precursor of most adenocarcinomas is clinically silent in up to 90% of cases. The symptomatology of Barrett oesophagus, when present, is that of gastro-oesophageal reflux {1011}. This is the condition where the early stages of neoplasia (intraepithelial and intramucosal neoplasia) should be sought.

Endoscopy
The endoscopic analysis of the squamocolumnar junction aims at the detection of columnar metaplasia in the distal oesophagus. At endoscopy, the squamocolumnar junction (Z-line) is in the thorax, just above the narrowed passage across the diaphragm. The anatomical landmarks in this area are treated in the chapter on tumours of the oesophagogastric junction.
If the length of the columnar lining in this distal oesophageal segment is ≥ 3 cm, it is termed a long type of Barrett metaplasia. When the length is < 3 cm, it is a short type. Single or multiple finger-like (1-3 cm) protrusions of columnar mucosa are classified as short type. In patients with short segment (< 3 cm) Barrett oesophagus the risk for developing adenocarcinoma is reported to be lower compared to those with long segment Barrett oesophagus {1720}.
As Barrett oesophagus is restricted to cases with histologically confirmed intestinal metaplasia, adequate tissue sampling is required.

Histopathology
Barrett epithelium is characterized by two different types of cells, i.e. goblet cells and columnar cells, and has also been termed 'specialized', 'distinctive' or Barrett metaplasia. The goblet cells stain positively with Alcian blue at low pH (2.5). The metaplastic epithelium has a flat or villiform surface, and is identical to gastric intestinal metaplasia of the incomplete type (type II or III). Rarely, foci of complete intestinal metaplasia (type I) with absorptive cells and Paneth cells may be found. The mucous glands beneath the surface epithelium and pits may also contain metaplastic epithelium. Recent studies suggest that the columnar metaplasia originates from multipotential cells located in intrinsic oesophageal glands {1429}.

Intraepithelial neoplasia in Barrett oesophagus
Macroscopy
Intraepithelial neoplasia generally has no distinctive gross features, and is detected by systematic sampling of a flat Barrett mucosa {634, 1573}. The area involved is variable, and the presence of multiple dysplastic foci is common {226, 1197}.
In some cases, intraepithelial neoplasia presents as one or several nodular masses resembling sessile adenomas. Rare dysplastic lesions have been considered true adenomas, with an expanding but localised growth resulting in a well demarcated interface with the surrounding tissue {1459}.

Microscopy
Epithelial atypia in Barrett mucosa is usually assessed according to the system

Table 1.02
Pattern of endoscopic ultrasound in oesophageal cancer. There are three hyper- and two hypoechoic layers; the tumour mass is hypoechoic.

T1	The 2nd hyperechoic layer (submucosa) is continuous
T2	The 2nd hyperechoic layer (submucosa) is interrupted The 3rd hyperechoic layer (adventitia) is continuous
T3	The 3rd hyperechoic layer (aventitia) is interrupted
T4	The hypoechoic tumour is continuous with adjacent structures

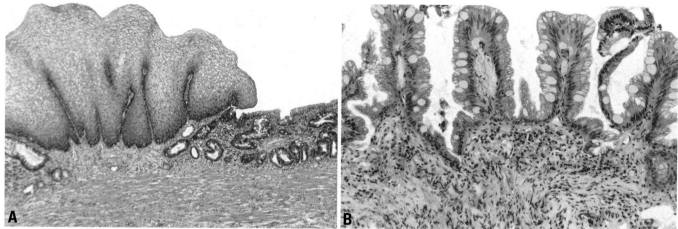

Fig. 1.23 Barrett oesophagus. **A** Haphazardly arranged glands (right) adjacent to hyperplastic squamous epithelium (left). **B** Goblet cells and columnar cells form villus-like structures over chronically inflamed stroma. There is no intraepithelial neoplasia.

devised for atypia in ulcerative colitis, namely: negative, positive or indefinite for intraepithelial neoplasia. If intraepithelial neoplasia is present, it should be classified as low-grade (synonymous with mild or moderate dysplasia) or high-grade (synonymous with severe dysplasia and carcinoma *in situ*) {1582, 1685}. The criteria used to grade intraepithelial neoplasia comprise cytological and architectural features {75}.

Negative for intraepithelial neoplasia
Usually, the lamina propria of Barrett mucosa contains a mild accompanying inflammatory infiltrate of mononuclear cells. There may be mild reactive changes with enlarged, hyperchromatic nuclei, prominence of nucleoli, and occasional mild stratification in the lower portion of the glands. However, towards the surface there is maturation of the epithelium with few or no abnormalities. These changes meet the criteria of atypia negative for intraepithelial neoplasia, and can usually be separated from low-grade intraepithelial neoplasia.

Atypia indefinite for intraepithelial neoplasia. One of the major challenges for the pathologist in Barrett oesophagus is the differentiation of intraepithelial neoplasia from reactive or regenerative epithelial changes. This is particularly difficult, sometimes even impossible, if erosions or ulcerations are present {1055}. In areas adjacent to erosions and ulcerations, the metaplastic epithelium may display villiform hyperplasia of the surface foveolae with cytological atypia and architectural disturbances. These abnormalities are usually milder than those observed in intraepithelial neoplasia. There is a normal expansion of the basal replication zone in regenerative epithelium *versus* intraepithelial neoplasia, where the proliferation shifts to more superficial portions of the gland {738}. If there is doubt as to whether reactive and regenerative changes or intraepithelial neoplasia is present in a biopsy, the category atypia indefinite for intraepithelial neoplasia is appropriate and a repeat biopsy after reflux control by medical acid suppression or anti-reflux therapy is indicated.

Low-grade and high-grade intraepithelial neoplasia. Intraepithelial neoplasia in Barrett metaplastic mucosa is defined as a neoplastic process limited to the epithelium {1582}. Its prevalence in Barrett mucosa is approximately 10%, and it develops only in the intestinal type metaplastic epithelium.
Cytological abnormalities typically extend to the surface of the mucosa. In low-grade intraepithelial neoplasia, there is decreased mucus secretion, nuclear pseudostratification confined to the lower half of the glandular epithelium, occasional mitosis, mild pleomorphism, and minimal architectural changes.
High-grade intraepithelial neoplasia shows marked pleomorphism and decrease of mucus secretion, frequent mitosis, nuclear stratification extending

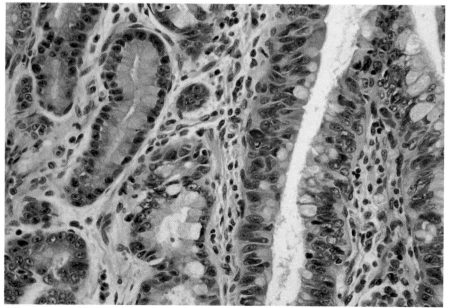

Fig. 1.24 Barrett oesophagus with low-grade intraepithelial neoplasia on the left and high-grade on the right. Note the numerous goblet cells showing a clear cytoplasmic mucous vacuole indenting the adjacent nucleus.

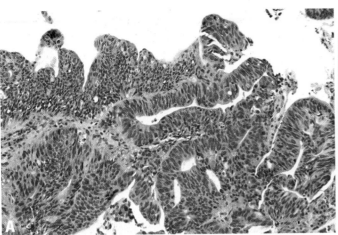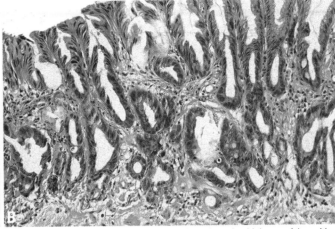

Fig. 1.25 High-grade intraepithelial neoplasia in Barrett oesophagus. **A** Marked degree of stratification with nuclei being present throughout the thickness of the epithelium. Foci of cribriform, back-to-back glands. **B** Highly atypical cells lining tubular structures.

to the upper part of the cells and glands, and marked architectural aberrations. The most severe architectural changes consist of a cribriform pattern that is a feature of high-grade intraepithelial neoplasia as long as the basement membrane of the neoplastic glands has not been disrupted. The diagnostic reproducibility of intraepithelial neoplasia is far from perfect; significant interobserver variation exists {1572}.

Adenocarcinoma

Symptoms and signs

Dysphagia is often the first symptom of advanced adenocarcinoma in the oesophagus. This may be associated with retrosternal or epigastric pain or cachexia.

Endoscopy

The endoscopic pattern of the early tumour stages may be that of a small polypoid adenomatous-like lesion, but more often it is flat, depressed, elevated or occult {1011, 1009}. Areas with high

grade intraepithelial neoplasia are often multicentric and occult. Therefore a systematic tissue sampling has been recommended when no abnormality is evident macroscopically {483}. The usual pattern of advanced adenocarcinoma at endoscopy is that of an axial, and often tight, stenosis in the distal third of the oesophagus; with a polypoid tumour, bleeding occurs at contact.

Radiology

This approach is still proposed in the primary diagnosis of oesophageal cancer when endoscopic access is not easily available {1058}. Today, barium studies are helpful mostly for the analysis of stenotic segments; they are less efficient than endoscopy for the detection of flat abnormalities. Computerised tomography will detect distant thoracic and abdominal metastases.

Endoscopic ultrasonography

At high frequency, some specificities in the echoic pattern of the mucosa and submucosa of the columnar lined oesophagus are displayed. However, the procedure is only suitable for the staging of tumours previously detected at endoscopy; the tumour is hypoechoic. Lymph nodes adjacent to the oesophageal wall can also be visualised by this technique {1614}.

Macroscopy

The majority of primary adenocarcinomas of the oesophagus arise in the lower third of the oesophagus within a segment of Barrett mucosa {1055}. Adjacent to the tumour, the typical salmon-pink mucosa

of Barrett oesophagus may be evident, especially in early carcinomas. In the early stages, the gross findings of Barrett adenocarcinoma may be subtle with irregular mucosal bumps or small plaques. At the time of diagnosis, most tumours are advanced with deep infiltration of the oesophageal wall. The advanced carcinomas are predominantly flat and ulcerated with only one third having a polypoid or fungating appearance. Occasionally, multifocal tumours

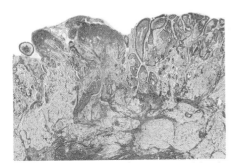

Fig. 1.26 Mucinous adenocarcinoma arising in Barrett oesophagus. Large mucinous lakes extend throughout the oesophageal wall.

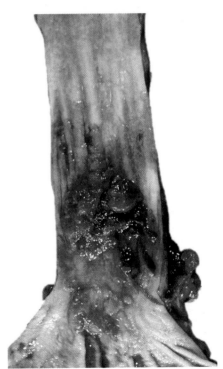

Fig. 1.27 Highly infiltrative adenocarcinoma in Barrett oesophagus (stage pT3), with extension into the cardia.

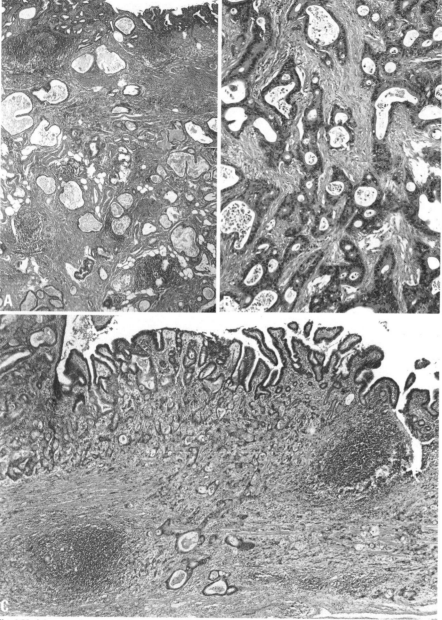

Fig. 1.28 Adenocarcinoma, tubular type. **A** Well differentiated, **B** moderately differentiated and **C** poorly differentiated.

The well differentiated tumours may pose a diagnostic problem in biopsy specimens because the infiltrating component may be difficult to recognize as invasive {1055} since Barrett mucosa often has irregular dispersed glands. Glandular structures are only slightly formed in poorly differentiated adenocarcinomas and absent in undifferentiated tumours. *Small cell carcinoma* may show foci of glandular differentiation. It is discussed in the chapter on endocrine neoplasms of the oesophagus.

Tumour spread and staging
Adenocarcinomas spread first locally and infiltrate the oesophageal wall. Distal spread to the stomach may occur. Extension through the oesophageal wall into adventitial tissue, and then into adjacent organs or tissues is similar to squamous cell carcinoma. Common sites of local spread comprise the mediastinum, tracheobronchial tree, lung, aorta, pericardium, heart and spine {1055, 1789}. Barrett associated adenocarcinoma metastasizes to para-oesophageal and paracardial lymph nodes, those of the lesser curvature of the stomach and the celiac nodes. Distant metastases occur late. The TNM classification used for SCC is applicable to Barrett adenocarcinoma and provides prognostically significant data {1945}.

Other carcinomas
Adenosquamous carcinoma
(ICD-O code: 8560/3)
This carcinoma has a significant squamous carcinomatous component that is intermingled with a tubular adenocarcinoma.

Mucoepidermoid carcinoma
(ICD-O code: 8430/3)
This rare carcinoma shows an intimate mixture of squamous cells, mucus secreting cells and cells of an intermediate type.

Adenoid cystic carcinoma
(ICD-O code: 8200/3)
This neoplasm is also infrequent and believed to arise, like the mucoepidermoid variant, from oesophageal glands {265, 2066}. Both lesions tend to be of salivary gland type, and small tumours may be confined to the submucosa. However, the ordinary oesophageal adenocarcinoma can also arise from ectopic gastric glands, or oesophageal glands {1204, 1055}.

may be present {1055, 1770}. The rare adenocarcinomas arising independently of Barrett oesophagus from ectopic gastric glands and oesophageal glands display predominantly ulceration and polypoid gross features, respectively. These tumours are also found in the upper and middle third of the oesophagus {265, 1204}, but are rare.

Histopathology
Adenocarcinomas arising in the setting of Barrett oesophagus are typically papillary and/or tubular. A few tumours are of the diffuse type and show rare glandular formations, and sometimes signet ring cells {1458, 1770}. Differentiation may produce endocrine cells, Paneth cells and squamous epithelium. Mucinous adenocarcinomas, i.e. tumours with more than 50% of the lesion consisting of mucin, also occur.

Grading
Most adenocarcinomas arising from Barrett mucosa are well or moderately differentiated {1458}, and display well formed tubular or papillary structures.

Genetic susceptibility

Several lines of evidence suggest that there is a genetic susceptibility to oesophageal adenocarcinoma arising from Barrett oesophagus. The almost exclusive occurrence of Barrett oesophagus in whites and its strong male predominance hint at the involvement of genetic factors {1605}. Several reports describe familial clustering of Barrett oesophagus, adenocarcinoma and reflux symptoms in up to three generations, with some families showing an autosomal dominant pattern of inheritance with nearly complete penetrance {470, 480, 482, 569, 861, 1537, 1610, 1959}. Although shared dietary or environmental factors in these families could play a role, the earlier age of onset of Barrett in some families suggests the influence of genetic factors {861}. The molecular factors that determine this genetic susceptibility are largely unknown and linkage analysis in families has not been reported. Recently, an association between a variant of the *GSTP1* (glutathione S-transferase P1) gene and Barrett oesophagus and adenocarcinoma has been demonstrated {1994}. GSTs are responsible for the detoxification of various carcinogens, and inherited differences in carcinogen detoxification capacity may contribute to the development of Barrett epithelium and adenocarcinoma.

Genetics

In Barrett oesophagus a variety of molecular genetic changes has been correlated with the metaplasia-dysplasia-carcinoma sequence (Fig. 1.21) {2091}. Prospective follow-up of lesions biopsied at endoscopy show that alterations in *TP53* and *CDKN2A* occur at early stages {112, 1337}.

TP53. In high-grade intraepithelial neoplasia a prevalence of *TP53* mutations of approximately 60% is found, similar to adenocarcinoma {789}. Mutation in one allele is often accompanied by loss of the other (17p13.1). Mutations occur in diploid cells and precede aneuploidy. The pattern of mutations differs significantly from that in squamous cell carcinomas. This is particularly evident for the high frequency of G:C>A:T transition mutations, which prevail in adenocarcinomas but are infrequent in SCC (Fig. 1.17).

CDKN2A. Alterations of *CDKN2A,* a locus on 9p21 encoding two distinct tumour suppressors, p16 and p19^{arf}

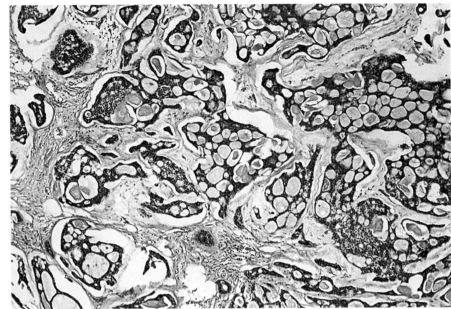

Fig. 1.29 Adenoid cystic carcinoma showing typical cribriform pattern resembling its salivary gland counterpart.

include hypermethylation of the p16 promotor and, more rarely, mutations and LOH {948}.

FHIT. Among other early changes in the premalignant stages of metaplasia are alterations of the transcripts of *FHIT*, a presumptive tumour suppressor gene spanning the common fragile site FRA3B {1222}.

LOH and gene amplification. A number of other loci are altered relatively late during the development of adenocarcinoma, with no obligate sequence of events. Prevalent changes (> 50%) include LOH on chromosomes 4 (long arm) and 5 (several loci including APC) and amplification of *ERBB2* {1266, 1264}.

Phenotypic changes in Barrett oesopha-

Table 1.03
Genes and proteins involved in carcinogenesis in Barrett oesophagus.

Factor	Comment
Tumour suppressor genes	
TP53	60% Mutation – high-grade intraepithelial neoplasia and carcinoma
APC	Late in intraepithelial neoplasia-carcinoma sequence
FHIT	Common, early abnormalities
CDKN2A (p16)	Hypermethylation common in intraepithelial neoplasia
Growth factor receptors	
CD95/APO/Fas	Shift to cytoplasm in carcinoma
EGFR	Expressed in 60% carcinomas, gene amplification
c-erbB2	Late in dysplasia-carcinoma sequence, gene amplification
Cell adhesion	
E-cadherin	Loss of expression in intraepithelial and invasive carcinoma
Catenins	Similar loss of expression to E-cadherin
Proteases	
UPA	Prognostic factor in carcinoma
Proliferation	
Ki-67	Abnormal distribution in high-grade intraepithelial neoplasia
Membrane trafficking	
rab11	High expression in low-grade intraepithelial neoplasia

gus include expansion of the Ki-67 proliferation compartment correlating with the degree of intraepithelial neoplasia {738}. Molecules involved in membrane trafficking such as rab11 have been reported to be specific for the loss of polarity seen in low-grade intraepithelial neoplasia {1566}. In invasive carcinoma, reduced expression of cadherin/catenin complex and increased expression of various proteases are detectable. Non-neoplastic Barrett oesophagus expresses the MUC2 but not the MUC1 mucin gene product, whereas neither is expressed in intraepithelial neoplasia in Barrett

oesophagus {298}. Invasive lesions exhibit variable expression of MUC1 and MUC2.

Prognostic factors

The major prognostic factors in adenocarcinoma of the oesophagus are the depth of mural invasion and the presence or absence of lymph node or distant metastasis {734, 1049, 1458, 1945}. Gross features and histological differentiation do not influence prognosis. The overall 5-year survival rate after surgery is less than 20% in most series including a majority of advanced carcinomas. The

survival rates are better in superficial (pT1) adenocarcinoma, ranging from 65% to 80% in different series {735, 1219}.

Since the stage at the time of diagnosis is the most important factor affecting outcome, endoscopic surveillance of Barrett patients with early detection of their adenocarcinomas, results in better prognosis in most cases {1995}.

Endocrine tumours of the oesophagus

C. Capella
E. Solcia
L.H. Sobin
R. Arnold

Definition

Endocrine tumours of the oesophagus are rare and include carcinoid (well differentiated endocrine neoplasm), small cell carcinoma (poorly differentiated endocrine carcinoma), and mixed endocrine-exocrine carcinoma.

ICD-O codes

Carcinoid	8240/3
Small cell carcinoma	8041/3
Mixed endocrine-exocrine carcinoma	8244/3

Epidemiology

In an analysis of 8305 carcinoid tumours of different sites, only 3 (0.04%) carcinoids of the oesophagus were reported {1251}. They represented 0.05% of all gastrointestinal carcinoids reported in this analysis and 0.02% of all oesophageal cancers. All cases were in males and presented at a mean age of 56 years {1251}. Small cell carcinoma occurs mainly in the sixth to seventh decade and is twice as common in males as females {190, 421, 765, 1026}. The reported frequencies among all oesophageal cancers were between 0.05% to 7.6 % {190, 421, 765, 1026}.

The few mixed endocrine-exocrine carcinomas were in males at the sixth decade {256, 301}.

Aetiological factors

Patients with small cell carcinomas often have a history of heavy smoking and one reported case was associated with long standing achalasia {93, 1539}. A case of combined adenocarcinoma and carcinoid occurred in a patient with a Barrett oesophagus {256}. Small cell carcinoma has also been associated with Barrett oesophagus {1678, 1813}.

Localization

Carcinoid tumours are typically located in the lower third of the oesophagus {1329, 1567, 1754}. Almost all small cell carcinomas occur in the distal half of the oesophagus {190, 421}.

Clinical features

Dysphagia, severe weight loss and sometimes chest pain are the main symptoms of endocrine tumours of the oesophagus. Patients with small cell carcinomas often present at an advanced stage {765, 1026}. Inappropriate antidiuretic hormone syndrome and hypercalcemia have been reported {421}. In addition, a case

of watery diarrhoea, hypokalaemia-achlor-hydria (WDHA) syndrome, due to ectopic production of VIP by a mixed-cell (squamous-small cell) carcinoma of the oesophagus has been described {2070}.

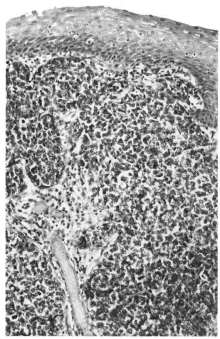

Fig. 1.30 Small cell carcinoma of the oesophagus.

Macroscopy

All reported oesophageal carcinoids were of large size (from 4 to 7 cm in diameter) and infiltrated deeply the oesophageal wall {1329, 1567, 1754}. Small cell carcinomas usually appear as fungating or ulcerated masses of large size, measuring from 4 to 14 cm in greatest diameter.

Histopathology

Carcinoid (well differentiated endocrine neoplasm)

All carcinoids so far reported in the literature have been described as deeply infiltrative tumours, with high mitotic rate and metastases {1329, 1567, 1754}. Microscopically, they are composed of solid nests of tumour cells that show positive stain for Grimelius and neuron-specific enolase {1567}, and characteristic membrane-bound neurosecretory granules at ultrastructural examination {1754}.

Small cell carcinoma (poorly differentiated endocrine carcinoma)

Small cell carcinoma of the oesophagus is indistinguishable from its counterpart in the lung according to histological and immunohistochemical features as well as clinical behaviour. The cells may be small with dark nuclei of round or oval shape and scanty cytoplasm, or be larger with more cytoplasm (intermediate cells) forming solid sheets and nests. There may be foci of squamous carcinoma, adenocarcinoma, and/or mucoepidermoid carcinoma, a finding that raises the possibility of an origin of tumour cells from pluripotent cells present in the squamous epithelium or ducts of the submucosal glands {190, 1887}. Argyrophylic granules can be demonstrated by Grimelius stain, and small dense-core granules are always detected by electron microscopy {781}.

Immunohistochemical reactions for neuron-specific enolase, synaptophysin, chromogranin and leu7 usually are positive and represent useful diagnostic markers {723}. Some cases have been associated with calcitonin and ACTH production {1272}.

Mixed endocrine-exocrine carcinoma

In the few reported cases {256, 301}, the tumours combined a gastrointestinal-type adenocarcinoma with the trabecular-acinar component of a carcinoid. In one case the carcinoid component was positive for Grimelius stain, Fontana argentaffin reaction and formaldehyde induced fluorescence for amines {301}.

Prognostic factors

Two of three oesophageal carcinoids from the analysis of 8305 cases of carcinoid tumours {1251} were associated with distant metastases and one {1567} of the three reported cases {1329, 1567, 1754} died 29 months after surgery.

The prognosis of small cell carcinoma of the oesophagus is poor, even when the primary growth is limited {190, 421}. The survival period is usually less than 6 months {816 and thus similar to that of patients with small cell carcinoma of the colon {765, 1026}. Multidrug chemotherapy may offer temporary remission {765, 816, 1026, 1678}.

Lymphoma of the oesophagus

A. Wotherspoon
A. Chott
R.D. Gascoyne
H.K. Müller-Hermelink

Definition

Primary lymphoma of the oesophagus is defined as an extranodal lymphoma arising in the oesophagus with the bulk of the disease localized to this site {796}. Contiguous lymph node involvement and distant spread may be seen but the primary clinical presentation is in the oesophagus with therapy directed at this site.

Clinical features

The oesophagus is the least common site of involvement with lymphoma in the digestive tract, accounting for less than 1% of lymphoma patients {1399}. Oesophageal involvement is usually secondary either from the mediastinum, from nodal disease or from a primary gastric location. Patients are frequently male and usually over 50 years old. Tumours involving the distal portion of the oesophagus may cause dysphagia {644}.

Histopathology

Primary oesophageal lymphomas may be of the large B-cell type or may be low-grade B-cell MALT lymphomas {1794}. MALT lymphomas show morphological and cytological features common to MALT lymphomas found elsewhere in the digestive tract. Lymphoid follicles are surrounded by a diffuse infiltrate of centrocyte-like (CCL) cells showing a variable degree of plasma cell differentiation. Infiltration of these cells into the overlying epithelium is usually seen. Characteristically the CCL cells express pan-B-cell markers CD20 and CD79a and they are negative for CD5 and CD10. They express bcl-2 protein and may be positive with antibodies to CD43. Due to the rarity of these lesions, molecular genetics data are not available.

In common with other sites in the digestive tract, secondary involvement of the oesophagus may occur in dissemination of any type of lymphoma.

Primary oesophageal T-cell lymphoma has been described but is exceedingly rare {547}.

Mesenchymal tumours of the oesophagus

M. Miettinen
J.Y. Blay
L.H. Sobin

Definition

A variety of rare benign and malignant mesenchymal tumours that arise in the oesophagus. Among these, tumours of smooth muscle or 'stromal' type are most common.

ICD-O codes

Leiomyoma	8890/0
Leiomyosarcoma	8890/3
Gastrointestinal stromal tumour (GIST)	8936/3
Granular cell tumour	9580/0
Rhabdomyosarcoma	8900/3
Kaposi sarcoma	9190/3

Classification

The morphological definitions of these lesions follow the WHO histological classification of soft tissue tumours {2086}. Stromal tumours are described in detail in the chapter on gastric mesenchymal tumours.

Epidemiology

Leiomyoma is the most common mesenchymal tumour of the oesophagus. It occurs in males at twice the frequency as females and has a median age distribution between 30 and 35 years {1712, 1228}. *Sarcomas* of the oesophagus accounted for 0.2% of malignant oesophageal tumours in SEER data from the United States from 1973 to 1987. Males were more frequently affected than females by nearly 2:1 {1928}. Adults between the 6th and 8th decades are primarily affected. Oesophageal stromal tumours show demographics similar to those of sarcomas {1228}.

Localization

Leiomyomas and *stromal tumours* are most frequent in the lower oesophagus and begin as intramural lesions. The larger tumours can extend to mediastinum and form a predominantly mediastinal mass. *Leiomyomatosis* forms worm-like intramural structures that may extend into the upper portion of the stomach.

Clinical features

Dysphagia is the usual complaint, but many leiomyomas and a small proportion of stromal tumours are asymptomatic and are incidentally detected by X-ray as mediastinal masses. Since most sarcomas project into the lumen, they are relatively easy to diagnose by endoscopy or imaging studies. The endoscopic pattern is that of a submucosal tumour with a swelling of a normal mucosa. Endoscopic ultrasound helps in determining the actual size of the tumour, its position in the oesophageal wall and its eventual position in the mediastinum. A CT scan of the mediastinum is then a useful compliment. Most tumours less than 3 cm in diameter are benign. Endoscopic tissue sampling (large biopsy or fine needle aspiration) is difficult and not very reliable for the assessment of malignancy.

Macroscopy

Leiomyomas vary in size from a few millimeters up to 10 cm in diameter (average 2-3 cm). They may be spherical, or when larger they can form sausage-like masses with a large longitudinal dimension or dumb-bell shaped masses with circular involvement {1712, 1228}. Large leiomyomas (over 0.5 kg) have been described {968}. *Sarcomas*, most of them representing malignant gastrointestinal stromal tumours (GISTs), are typically multinodular or less commonly plaque-like masses resembling sarcomas of the soft tissues. Many oesophageal sarcomas protrude into the mediastinum.

Histopathology

Leiomyoma is composed of bland spindle cells and shows low or moderate cellularity and slight if any mitotic activity. There may be focal nuclear atypia. The cells have eosinophilic, fibrillary, often clumped cytoplasm. Eosinophilic granulocytes and spherical calcifications are sometimes present. Leiomyomas are typically globally positive for desmin and smooth muscle actin, and are negative for CD34 and CD117 (KIT) {1228}.

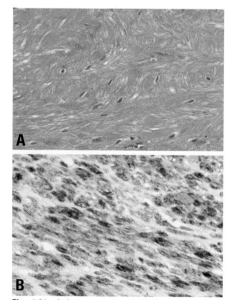

Fig. 1.31 Leiomyoma of oesophagus. **A** Haematoxylin and eosin stain. **B** Immunoreactivity for desmin.

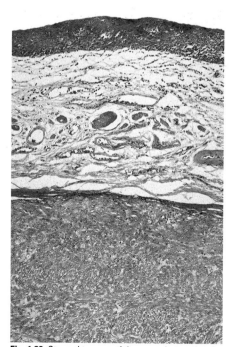

Fig. 1.32 Stromal tumour of the oesophagus, involving the oesophageal muscle layer beneath a normal mucosa.

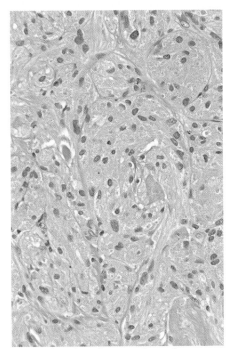

Fig. 1.33 Granular cell tumour of oesophagus.

Leiomyosarcoma, a malignant tumour featuring differentiated smooth muscle cells, is rare in the oesophagus. In a recent series, such tumours comprised 4% of all combined smooth muscle and stromal tumours. They were large tumours that presented in older adults, and all patients died of disease. Diagnosis is based on demonstration of smooth muscle differentiation by α-smooth muscle actin, desmin or both, and lack of KIT expression {1228}.

Stromal tumours (GISTs) are rare in the oesophagus, and comprise 20-30% of the combined cases of smooth muscle and stromal tumours. Like elsewhere in the digestive system, they predominantly occur in older adults between the 6th and 8th decades; oesophageal stromal tumours may have a male predominance. Most oesophageal examples are spindle cell tumours, and a minority are epithelioid. Oesophageal GISTs are identical with their gastric counterparts by their positivity for KIT and CD34, variable reactivity for smooth muscle actin and general negativity for desmin. Most are clinically malignant, and commonly develop liver metastases. The oesophageal tumours analyzed to date have shown similar *c-kit* mutations (exon 11) as observed in gastric and intestinal GISTs {1228}. The pathological features are described with gastric GISTs.

Granular cell tumours are usually detected endoscopically as nodules or small sessile polyps predominantly in the distal oesophagus {1216, 7}. Benign behaviour is the rule, but a case of malignant oesophageal granular cell tumour has been reported. The tumours are usually small, up to 1-2 cm in diameter, and are grossly yellow, firm nodules. Histologically they are composed of sheets of oval to polygonal cells with a small central nucleus and abundant granular slightly basophilic cytoplasm. This is due to extensive accumulation of lysosomes filled with lamellar material. Granular cell tumours are typically PAS- and S100-protein positive and negative for desmin, actin, CD34 and KIT. Tumours that encroach upon the mucosa may elicit a pseudocarcinomatous squamous hyperplasia {862, 1710}.

Rhabdomyosarcoma has been reported in older adult patients in distal oesophagus. A few well-documented cases have shown features similar to embryonal rhabdomyosarcoma {2002}. Demonstration of skeletal muscle differentiation by the presence of cross-striations, electron microscopy, or immunohistochemistry is required for the diagnosis.

Synovial sarcoma has been reported in children and in older adults. These tumours usually present as polypoid masses in the proximal oesophagus {168, 149}.

Kaposi sarcoma may appear as a mucosal or less commonly more extensive mural lesion, usually in HIV-positive patients. Histologically typical are spindle cells with vascular slit formations and scattered PAS-positive globules. The tumour cells are positive for CD31 and CD34.

Grading

Histological grading follows the systems commonly used for soft tissue tumours. Mitotic activity is the main criterion for grading stromal sarcomas and leiomyosarcomas, namely those tumours with over 10 mitoses per 10 HPF are considered high-grade.

Genetics

Somatic deletions and gene rearrangements involving the genes encoding alpha5 and 6 chains of collagen type IV have been described in oesophageal leiomyomatosis associated with Alport syndrome {1704, 1982} and in sporadic

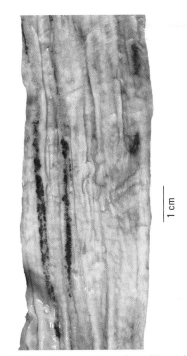

Fig. 1.34 Kaposi sarcoma in a patient with acquired immunodeficiency syndrome.

leiomyoma {683}, whereas these tumours do not have *c-kit* gene mutations commonly found in GISTs {1018}. Comparative genomic hybridization studies have shown that oesophageal leiomyomas do not have losses of chromosome 14, as often seen in GIST, but instead have gains in chromosome 5 {450, 1664}. Oesophageal stromal tumours show similar *c-kit* mutations as observed in gastric and intestinal GISTs (see stomach mesenchymal tumours) {1228}.

Kaposi sarcoma is positive for human herpesvirus 8 by PCR.

Prognosis

The prognosis of oesophageal sarcomas, like carcinomas, is largely dependent on the size, depth of invasion, and presence or absence of metastasis.

Secondary tumours and melanoma of the oesophagus

G. Ilyés
A. Kádár
N.J. Carr

Secondary tumours

Definition
Tumours of the oesophagus that originate from but are discontinuous with a primary tumour elsewhere in the oesophagus or an extra-oesophageal neoplasm.

Incidence
Metastatic spread to the oesophagus is uncommon. An unusually high frequency (6.1% of autopsy cases) was reported from Japan {1249}.

Origin of metastases
The concept of intramural metastasis in oesophageal squamous cell carcinoma is discussed in the chapter on squamous cell carcinoma of the oesophagus. Neoplasms of neighbouring organs such as pharynx or gastric cardia {714} can spread to the oesophagus via lymphatics. Haematogenous metastases from any primary localization may occur. Reported primary sites include thyroid {335}, lung {1416, 1249}, breast {2143, 1249, 545}, skin {1569, 1203}, kidney {1956}, prostate {1318} and ovary {1249}.

Localization
The most common site of involvement is the middle third of the oesophagus.

Clinical features
The leading symptom is dysphagia, whereas achalasia and upper gastrointestinal bleeding with anemia are unusual {545}. Barium swallow examination, endoscopy, computed tomography and magnetic resonance imaging demonstrate in most cases a submucosal tumour, but any aspect resembling a primary oesophageal carcinoma may be observed {545, 1318, 714}.

Histopathology and predictive factors
Submucosal localization without invasion of the mucosa is characteristic for a metastasis. Early metastases of gastric and oesophageal tumours into the oesophagus may be local indicators of systemic spread {896, 714}. The presence of metastasis in the oesophagus is a sign of poor prognosis, but the outcome is much better when the primary tumour growth rate is slow, and when other metastases are excluded {1416, 1249}.

Melanoma

ICD-O Code   8720/3

Malignant melanoma in the oesophagus is much more commonly metastatic than primary. Primary oesophageal melanomas are usually polypoid and are clinically aggressive lesions {400, 353}. They are believed to arise from a zone of atypical junctional proliferation of melanocytes and such a proliferation is often present adjacent to the invasive tumour, although it may not be observed in advanced disease. The histology of the invasive component is indistinguishable from cutaneous melanoma {409}. Growth is typically expansile rather than infiltrative.

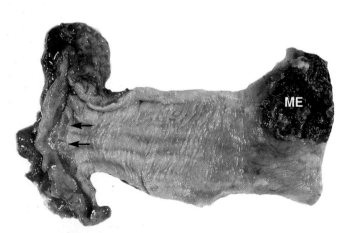

Fig. 1.35 Primary melanoma of the oesophagus (ME). The gastro-oesophageal junction is on the left (arrows).

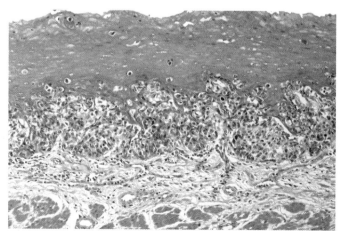

Fig. 1.36 Primary malignant melanoma of the distal oesophagus. Zone of atypical junctional proliferation of melanocytes located adjacent to the invasive tumour. This supports the diagnosis of a primary melanoma.

Contents

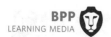

Introduction to the course

Syllabus overview

This unit is about the key aspects of taxation that affect UK taxpayers. It covers income tax, National Insurance (NI), capital gains tax and inheritance tax.

This unit provides students with the underpinning theory on taxation, such as what makes for a fair and equitable taxation system. Students then explore three core areas of income that contribute to a taxpayer's income tax liability: employment income, income from investments and income from property. Deductions and reliefs that apply to this income are then covered, so that students can compute the net income tax payable or reclaimable for a UK taxpayer.

The unit covers NI as applicable to employment income, together with the key principles that are part of capital gains tax and inheritance tax.

Students are also expected to demonstrate their knowledge and understanding of how UK taxpayers can minimise their tax liability legally. For example, investing in a new individual savings account (NISA) will ensure that interest on the investment will be exempt from tax, whereas an investment in a building society will usually give rise to a tax implication. The ethical issues that surround this complex area will also be considered.

Taking all areas together, students will gain knowledge and understanding of all key areas of UK tax that can affect an individual UK taxpayer.

Personal Tax is an optional unit.

Assessment type	Marking type	Duration of exam
Computer based assessment	Partially computer / partially human marked	2.5 hours

Learning outcomes		Weighting
1	Analyse the theories, principles and rules that underpin taxation systems	10%
2	Calculate a UK taxpayer's total income	28%
3	Calculate income tax and National Insurance (NI) contributions payable by a UK taxpayer	23%
4	Account for capital gains tax	27%
5	Discuss the basics of inheritance tax	12%

AAT

Personal Tax FA 2016

AQ 2016 Level 4

Course Book

For assessments from 1 January 2017

Second edition December 2016

ISBN 9781 5097 1075 1
ISBN (for internal use only) 9781 5097 1082 9

British Library Cataloguing-in-Publication Data
A catalogue record for this book is available from the British Library

Published by

BPP Learning Media Ltd
BPP House, Aldine Place
142-144 Uxbridge Road
London W12 8AA

www.bpp.com/learningmedia

Printed in the United Kingdom by Wheatons Exeter Ltd
Hennock Road
Marsh Barton
Exeter
EX2 8RP

Your learning materials, published by BPP Learning Media Ltd, are printed on paper obtained from traceable sustainable sources.

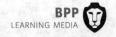

Assessment structure

2.5 hours duration

Competency is 70%

A significant amount of tax information is provided to you in the assessment. This is reproduced in this book in the *Reference material and tax tables* section.

At the time of writing the only guidance available about the assessment structure are the two sample assessments available on the AAT website. These two assessments both follow the same structure (outlined in the table below), and under previous syllabi the live assessment always followed the same structure as the relevant AAT sample assessment for that syllabus.

*Note that this is only a guideline as to what might come up. The format and content of each task may vary from what we have listed below.

The sample assessments both consisted of 13 tasks.

Task	Content	Max marks	Chapter ref	Study complete
Task 1	**Professional conduct – ethics** Written task, human marked	10	1 The tax and ethical framework	
Task 2	**Benefits in kind** Calculation of car and fuel benefits	8	4 Employment income	
Task 3	**Benefits in kind** Calculation of other benefits	8	4 Employment income	
Task 4	**Investment income** Calculation of taxable investment income from interest and dividends and the tax thereon including exempt income	6	6 Taxable income	
Task 5	**Property income** Calculation of taxable rental income and allowable expenditure for a number of different properties	6	5 Property income	

Task	Content	Max marks	Chapter ref	Study complete
Task 6	**Computation of taxable income and tax thereon** Assessed via free text box and human marked in live assessment. Requirement to list out net income, deduct personal allowance and calculate tax	12	6 Taxable income 7 Calculation of income tax	
Task 7	**National Insurance** Calculation of National Insurance Contributions	4	2 National insurance	
Task 8	**Sundry issues** This tested a number of separate areas: • Exempt income • Benefits • Tax planning • Personal pension contributions	7	4 Employment income 6 Taxable income 7 Calculation of income tax	
Task 9	**Basics of capital gains tax** This task required calculations for a number of different disposals testing chattels rules, connected parties, PPR, exempt assets and part disposals	10	8 Chargeable gains 10 Principal Private Residence	
Task 10	**Taxation of share disposal** Assessed by free text box and human marked. Rights and bonus issues were tested.	10	9 Share disposals	

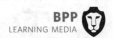

Task	Content	Max marks	Chapter ref		Study complete
Task 11	**Capital gains tax payable** Question required calculation of capital gains tax payable for a number of taxpayers with different income levels. Also, dealing with capital losses	7	8	Chargeable gains	
Task 12	**Inheritance tax** Multipart question testing several inheritance tax rules	6	3	Inheritance tax	
Task 13	**Inheritance tax** Detailed death tax on lifetime gifts and death estate calculation. Assessed by free text area and human marked	6	3	Inheritance tax	

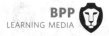

Skills bank

Our experience of preparing students for this type of assessment suggests that to obtain competency, you will need to develop a number of key skills.

What do I need to know to do well in the assessment?

This unit is one of the optional Level 4 units. To be successful in the assessment you need to be able to:

- Calculate employment income including benefits in kind
- Calculate property income
- Produce a schedule showing income from all sources including investment income
- Calculate the personal allowance a taxpayer is entitled to
- Calculate income tax and national insurance for a wide range of taxpayers including those who have given money to charity or paid into a pension
- Calculate the chargeable gains arising in different scenarios including the disposal of shares and private residences
- Calculate inheritance tax

Assumed knowledge

No prior knowledge of tax is expected but if you have worked in tax or previously studied the *Business Tax* unit then you will have an immediate advantage.

Assessment style

In the assessment you will complete tasks by:

1. Entering narrative by selecting from drop down menus of narrative options known as **picklists**

2. Using **drag and drop** menus to enter narrative

3. Typing in numbers, known as **gapfill** entry

4. Entering **ticks**

5. Entering **dates** by selecting from a calendar

6. Writing written explanations in a very basic word processing environment which has limited editing and no spelling or grammar checking functionality

7. Entering detailed calculations in a very basic spreadsheet environment that has limited editing functionality and will not perform calculations for you

You must familiarise yourself with the style of the online questions and the AAT software before taking the assessment. As part of your revision, login to the **AAT website** and attempt their **online practice assessment.**

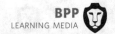

Introduction to the assessment

The question practice you do will prepare you for the format of tasks you will see in the *Personal Taxation* assessment. It is also useful to familiarise yourself with the introductory information you **may** be given at the start of the assessment.

1   As you revise, use the **BPP Passcards** to consolidate your knowledge. They are a pocket-sized revision tool, perfect for packing in that last-minute revision.

2   Attempt as many tasks as possible in the **Question Bank**. There are plenty of assessment-style tasks which are excellent preparation for the real assessment.

3   Always **check** through your own answers as you will in the real assessment, before looking at the solutions in the back of the Question Bank.

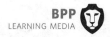

Key to icons

	Key term	A key definition which is important to be aware of for the assessment
	Formula to learn	A formula you will need to learn as it will not be provided in the assessment
	Formula provided	A formula which is provided within the assessment and generally available as a pop-up on screen
	Activity	An example which allows you to apply your knowledge to the technique covered in the Course Book. The solution is provided at the end of the chapter
	Illustration	A worked example which can be used to review and see how an assessment question could be answered
	Assessment focus point	A high priority point for the assessment
	Open book reference	Where use of an open book will be allowed for the assessment
	Real life examples	A practical real life scenario

AAT qualifications

The material in this book may support the following AAT qualifications:

AAT Professional Diploma in Accounting Level 4, AAT Professional Diploma in Accounting at SCQF Level 8 and Certificate: Accounting (Level 5 AATSA).

Supplements

From time to time we may need to publish supplementary materials to one of our titles. This can be for a variety of reasons, from a small change in the AAT unit guidance to new legislation coming into effect between editions.

You should check our supplements page regularly for anything that may affect your learning materials. All supplements are available free of charge on our supplements page on our website at:

www.bpp.com/learning-media/about/students

Improving material and removing errors

There is a constant need to update and enhance our study materials in line with both regulatory changes and new insights into the assessments.

From our team of authors BPP appoints a subject expert to update and improve these materials for each new edition.

Their updated draft is subsequently technically checked by another author and from time to time non-technically checked by a proof reader.

We are very keen to remove as many numerical errors and narrative typos as we can but given the volume of detailed information being changed in a short space of time we know that a few errors will sometimes get through our net.

We apologise in advance for any inconvenience that an error might cause. We continue to look for new ways to improve these study materials and would welcome your suggestions. Please feel free to contact our AAT Head of Programme at nisarahmed@bpp.com if you have any suggestions for us.

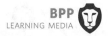

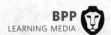

The tax and ethical framework

Learning outcomes

1	Analyse the theories, principles and rules that underpin taxation systems
1.1	**Evaluate the objectives and functions of taxation** • The principles underpinning tax systems • The features of tax systems, including tax bases and structures • How to compare progressive, regressive and proportional tax criteria used in evaluating a tax system
1.2	**Differentiate between tax planning, tax avoidance and tax evasion** • Definitions of tax planning, tax avoidance and tax evasion • Ethical implications of avoidance and evasion • Requirements to report suspected tax evasion under current legislation
1.3	**Discuss the roles and responsibilities of a taxation practitioner** • AAT's expectations of its members, as set out in the *AAT Code of Professional Ethics* • Principles of confidentiality, as applied in taxation situations • How to deal with clients and third parties
1.4	**Discuss residence and domicile** • The definitions of residence and domicile • The impact that each of these has on the taxation position of a UK taxpayer

Assessment context

Task 1 of the initial AAT sample assessment required you to discuss the implications of an ethical issue whereby you were presented with evidence that one of your clients was in receipt income that they had failed to advise you of. This was a 10-mark task that would be human marked in the live assessment.

Qualification context

Professional ethics are vital for a member of the AAT. The tax knowledge in this chapter is useful background in the *Business Tax* course.

Business context

A tax practitioner needs to know the duties and obligations that they owe to their client, the tax authorities and the Government.

A tax practitioner needs to know and understand the detailed tax rules.

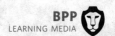

Chapter overview

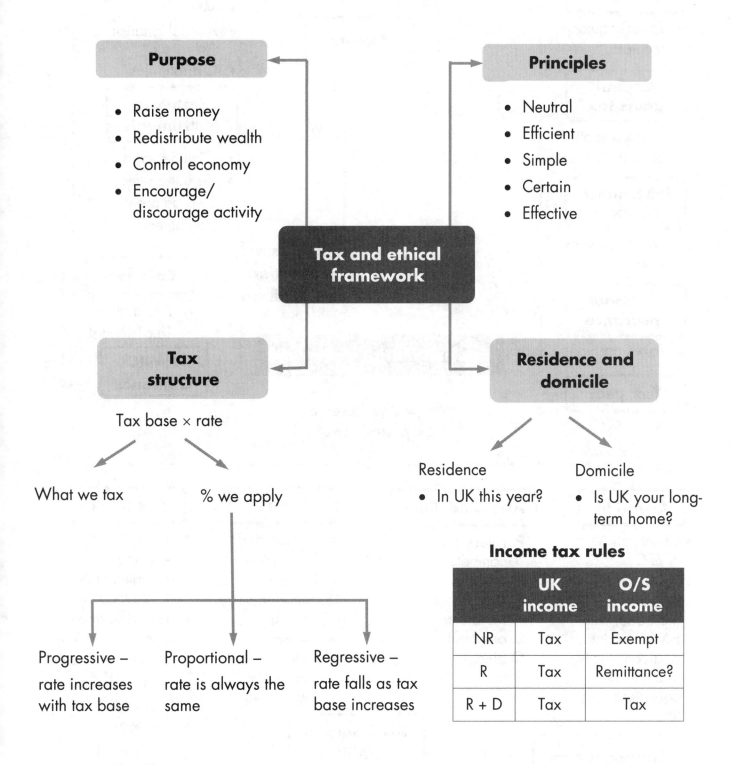

Purpose

- Raise money
- Redistribute wealth
- Control economy
- Encourage/ discourage activity

Principles

- Neutral
- Efficient
- Simple
- Certain
- Effective

Tax and ethical framework

Tax structure

Tax base × rate

What we tax

% we apply

Progressive – rate increases with tax base

Proportional – rate is always the same

Regressive – rate falls as tax base increases

Residence and domicile

Residence
- In UK this year?

Domicile
- Is UK your long-term home?

Income tax rules

	UK income	O/S income
NR	Tax	Exempt
R	Tax	Remittance?
R + D	Tax	Tax

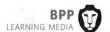

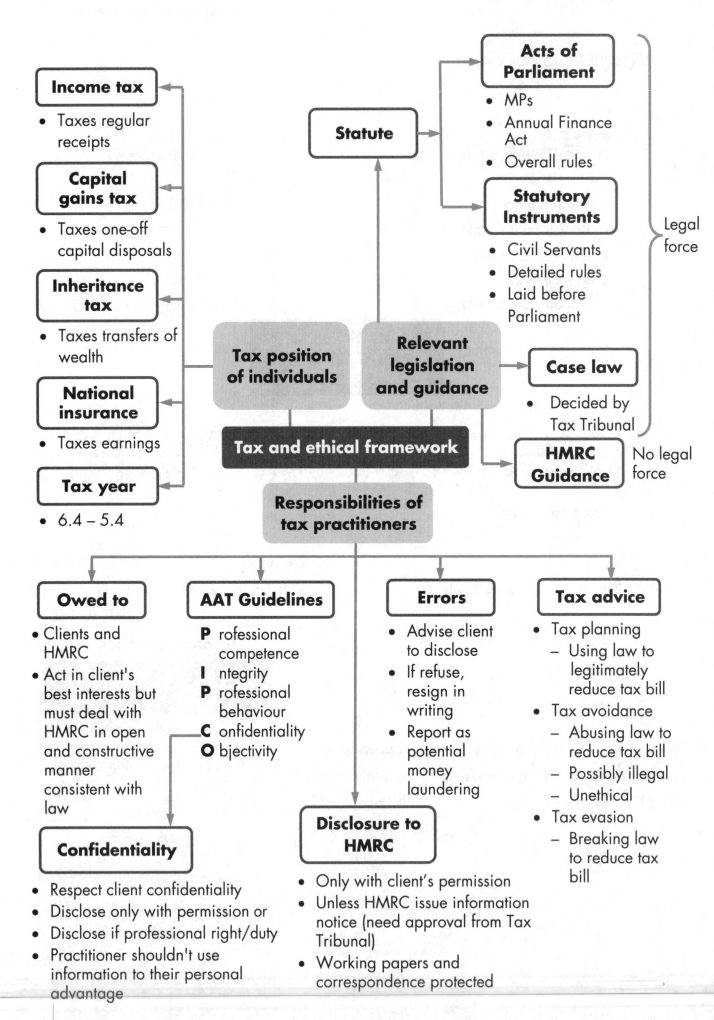

Income tax
- Taxes regular receipts

Capital gains tax
- Taxes one-off capital disposals

Inheritance tax
- Taxes transfers of wealth

National insurance
- Taxes earnings

Tax year
- 6.4 – 5.4

Statute

Acts of Parliament
- MPs
- Annual Finance Act
- Overall rules

Statutory Instruments
- Civil Servants
- Detailed rules
- Laid before Parliament

Legal force

Tax position of individuals

Relevant legislation and guidance

Case law
- Decided by Tax Tribunal

HMRC Guidance
No legal force

Tax and ethical framework

Responsibilities of tax practitioners

Owed to
- Clients and HMRC
- Act in client's best interests but must deal with HMRC in open and constructive manner consistent with law

AAT Guidelines
- **P** rofessional competence
- **I** ntegrity
- **P** rofessional behaviour
- **C** onfidentiality
- **O** bjectivity

Errors
- Advise client to disclose
- If refuse, resign in writing
- Report as potential money laundering

Tax advice
- Tax planning
  - Using law to legitimately reduce tax bill
- Tax avoidance
  - Abusing law to reduce tax bill
  - Possibly illegal
  - Unethical
- Tax evasion
  - Breaking law to reduce tax bill

Confidentiality
- Respect client confidentiality
- Disclose only with permission or
- Disclose if professional right/duty
- Practitioner shouldn't use information to their personal advantage

Disclosure to HMRC
- Only with client's permission
- Unless HMRC issue information notice (need approval from Tax Tribunal)
- Working papers and correspondence protected

Introduction

This chapter introduces you to some key background principles which will underlie all of your taxation studies and ethical principles that are vital to a tax practitioner working in the real world.

1 The objectives and functions of taxation

1.1 The purpose of taxation

Governments will collect taxation for a number of reasons:

The primary reason will be **to raise money for the government** to use in **providing infrastructure** such as roads **and services** such as the National Health Service.

Taxes can also be used as a means as **redistributing wealth** from rich to poor ensuring poorer people have an adequate standard of living and access to vital services.

Taxes can also be used to **control the economy**. In times of recession, taxes are cut to encourage people to spend money and stimulate the economy. In times of boom, taxes are raised to discourage people from spending money and causing the economy to overheat and crash.

Taxes can also be used to **encourage and discourage various types of activity**, for example the government wants us to save for our old age so we are not dependent on the state so paying into a pension saves you tax. Smoking will be harmful for you in the long run causing costs to the National Health Service so the government taxes it, this results in higher prices for consumers discouraging them from smoking.

1.2 Principles of taxation

There are a number of principles that should be considered when creating a tax system:

Generally, taxation should be **neutral** if possible. This means that the tax paid should not discourage or encourage taxpayers from taking a particular course of action. Also the government should not favour one business activity over another so different industries should not pay tax at different rates. Clearly this will not always be the case. As noted above often the government will use the tax system to influence the decisions people make.

Taxes should be **efficient**, this means the administration of the tax system should not cost an excessive amount otherwise the government will lose much of the revenue it raises before it has the chance to use if for the purposes for which it was collected.

Taxes should be **simple** and **certain**. This means they are easy to understand and calculate. If the rules are not simple taxpayers may be exposed to penalties because they have misunderstood the rules and not paid the right amount of tax which would seem unfair if this is no fault of their own. Conversely, complex tax rules provide greater scope for avoidance (see later). If tax rules are not certain then people cannot adequately plan their financial affairs. For example how could you decide whether to accept either a pay rise or use of a company car if you did not know how each would be taxed?

Taxes should be **effective**, collecting the money the government needs when they need it.

Taxes should be perceived as being **fair** or **equitable**. This is normally understood to mean that they should be based on the taxpayer's ability to pay.

1.3 Tax bases and structures

The **tax structure** of the country is essentially the way the tax system has been set up. At a simple level an amount (**the tax base**) will be taxed by multiplying it by a percentage (**the tax rate**). Governments will clearly have a lot of leeway to decide what is to be taxed and at what rate.

We will be studying the following UK taxes:

Key term

Income tax	The tax base here is income received by individuals (receipts which are expected to recur, for example the monthly receipt of a salary or rent received from an investment property). The tax rate will vary with the levels of income.
Capital gains tax	The tax base here is capital gains made by individuals (one-off profits on disposal of capital items, for example the sale of an investment property). The tax rate will vary with levels of income and the size of the gain.
National Insurance	The tax base here is earnings made by an individual from employment or self-employment (we are only concerned with employment rules in this module). The tax rate will vary with levels of earnings.
Inheritance tax	The tax base here is the value of wealth transferred by an individual. The tax rate varies depending on the amount of wealth transferred.

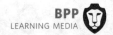

1.4 The rate of tax

When setting the rate of tax a government can choose between three different models:

Key term

Progressive	The tax rate here increases as the amount to be taxed (tax base) increases. This is usually perceived as being the fairest model.
Regressive	The tax rate here decreases as the amount to be taxed increases. This is usually perceived as being the unfairest model.
Proportional	The tax rate is always the same regardless of the level of income.

Most tax rates in the UK are progressive. For example, with income tax, no tax is paid on the first £11,000 of income then if the income is **non-savings** (see later) income tax is paid at 20%, then 40% then 45% as income increases.

Value Added Tax (VAT) (a tax not on your syllabus but you will have had experience of this in your day-to-day life) appears to be proportional as everyone pays 20% regardless of their level of income. However, there is an argument that this is a regressive tax as it is only levied on expenditure and poorer people will spend a greater proportion of their income than richer people. Poorer people are therefore paying a greater proportion of their income out as tax than richer people.

Note that you will be provided with much of this information in the reference material available in the assessment (and in the back of this Course Book).

2 The UK tax system

2.1 Her Majesty's Revenue & Customs

Taxes in the UK are administered by **Her Majesty's Revenue & Customs (HMRC)**.

2.2 Tax year

Key term

Tax year	This runs from 6 April to the following 5 April. It is also known as the **fiscal year** or the **year of assessment**. Tax is calculated on the income earned, wealth transferred and gains realised in the tax year.

The year of assessment 2016/17 runs from 6 April 2016 to 5 April 2017.

Some taxpayers will have to complete a tax return and pay tax under the self-assessment system. However, most taxpayers will have all their tax deducted at source. There is therefore no requirement for these taxpayers to complete a return.

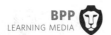

2.3 Legislation

The Government creates tax law. Tax laws consist of:

- **Acts of Parliament** – These are created via MPs debating in Parliament. There are a number of Acts that give the main rules for each of the UK taxes. These are updated each year by the annual **Finance Act**. Periodically they will be rewritten from scratch.

- **Statutory Instruments (SI)** – These are created by civil servants acting on behalf of the **Chancellor of the Exchequer**. They include the detailed rules for the operation of UK taxes. An SI will be laid before Parliament and becomes law if no objections are raised.

2.4 Case law

A taxpayer and HMRC may disagree over the interpretation of the **legislation**. Such disagreements will be heard by the **Tax Tribunal**. Once a decision has been reached, this has the force of law so all future taxpayers and HMRC officers must follow the decision.

2.5 HMRC guidance

HMRC publishes a range of guidance material to advise taxpayers as to how it interprets the law. HMRC guidance does not have legal force and could be challenged in court by a taxpayer.

3 Residence and domicile

Taxpayers are taxed in the UK with reference to their residence and domicile status.

3.1 Definitions

Key term

Residence	This is effectively a short-term test – is the taxpayer in the UK in a particular tax year?
Domicile	This is a long-term test – is the UK the taxpayer's real home?

It is relatively easy to lose or gain residence by coming to the UK or leaving it.

Domicile is a general law concept. If you were born in the UK, have lived here for most of your life, or are now living here permanently, this is a good indication that you are domiciled in the UK. However, many situations are more complex than this. There are three types of domicile: domicile of origin, domicile of dependence, and domicile of choice. You normally acquire a domicile of origin from your father when you are born, this means that even though you are born in the UK, you may not necessarily be UK domiciled. Until the age of 16, your domicile will follow the person on whom you are legally dependent, for example your father. You have the legal capacity to acquire a new domicile at the age of 16. However, to acquire a domicile of choice you must leave your current country of domicile and settle in another country permanently or indefinitely.

The test of residence is complex and you are not required to know the details. Generally though a taxpayer will be resident in the UK if they are present in the UK for more than half the tax year, their only home is in the UK or they carry out full time work in the UK.

3.2 Impact of the rules

3.2.1 Income tax

A taxpayer who is resident and domiciled in the UK pays tax in the UK on their worldwide income. This means they pay tax on all their income regardless as to where it is earned.

A taxpayer who is resident but not domiciled in the UK automatically pays tax in the UK on the income earned in the UK. Any income earned outside the UK may be subject to the remittance basis, this means it is only taxed in the UK if the taxpayer brings it into the UK. If the income is left outside the UK it is not subject to UK tax. The rules on claiming the remittance basis are complex and outside the scope of your assessment.

A non-resident individual only pays tax on income made in the UK. Income earned overseas cannot be taxed in the UK regardless as to whether it is brought into the UK or not

Illustration 1: Residence rules

Alan and Marie-Claude live in France. They both come to work in the UK. Alan was originally born in the UK and has retained ownership of his house in the UK. Marie-Claude was born in France and has always lived there.

Both receive rental income from letting out their French homes while they are working in the UK. The rental income is left in a French bank.

Both Alan and Marie-Claude will pay tax in the UK on their UK employment income.

Alan will have to pay tax on the French rental income in the UK because he is resident in the UK (he works in the UK) and domiciled in the UK (he was born in the UK and has retained his house in the UK).

Marie-Claude will probably not pay tax in the UK on the French rental income because although she is resident in the UK (she works in the UK) she is domiciled in France (she was born there and does not appear to have made steps to make the UK her permanent home). She will therefore be subject to the remittance basis and will only be taxed on the overseas income if she brings it into the UK.

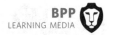

3.2.2 Income tax summary

	UK income	Overseas income
Not resident	Taxable	Exempt
Resident	Taxable	Remittance basis available
Resident and domiciled	Taxable	Taxable

3.2.3 Other taxes

We will consider the impact of residence and domicile on other taxes in the relevant chapters of this book.

4 Tax planning, tax avoidance and tax evasion

Nobody wants to pay tax! As a tax adviser your client will expect you to help them reduce their tax bill if possible. This is a complex area for an adviser because there are legal ways to reduce a tax bill encouraged by the government and illegal ways prevented by law and a grey area between the two.

Clearly as an adviser you should be helping your client but not breaking the law. These complex areas are addressed in the *Professional conduct in relation to taxation* section that follows.

4.1 Tax planning

This is perfectly legal and involves using the rules to reduce your tax bill in the way that they were intended for. For example paying into a pension scheme would reduce your tax bill.

The government accepts that everyone is entitled to structure their financial affairs in such a way that their tax bill is legally reduced to as little as possible.

4.2 Tax avoidance

On the face of it this appears permissible but is fraught with legal and ethical complications. It involves using the rules to reduce your tax bill in a way not intended by the government. You may not be breaking the law but you may be 'bending the rules' or exploiting 'a loophole'. By this we mean the actual words used in the relevant tax legislation may appear to permit you do something but it is clear that this was not the intention of the government when the law was written.

The taxpayer's reading of the law could be challenged by HMRC in court. If the judge does not agree with the taxpayer's interpretation then the avoidance will fail and the perpetrator will have to pay the avoided tax.

Often a taxpayer will have to engage in 'artificial transactions' when pursuing tax avoidance. This means that they are doing something purely to obtain a tax advantage, there can be no other reason for the transaction.

In the UK such artificial transactions can be set aside by the government making the tax avoidance ineffective.

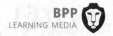

Illustration 2: Tax avoidance?

Dave is self-employed. His wife Doris works for him. Dave pays her £11,000 a year for the work she does. Does this represent tax avoidance?

This could represent tax avoidance or tax planning. It makes sense to have Doris work for the business as by paying her £11,000 this reduces the taxable profits of the business thereby reducing Dave's tax bill. If Doris has no other income this £11,000 would be covered by her personal allowance and she would pay no tax. This appears to be effective tax planning saving them money as a couple.

However, the key issues here would be: does Doris genuinely work for the business and does Dave pay her a commercial rate?

If she does not genuinely work for the business then this is avoidance and HMRC will set the whole transaction aside. Dave will be taxed on the £11,000.

If she is paid more than Dave would have paid someone else to do the same work then this is also avoidance. HMRC will set aside the excessive amount and Dave will be taxed on it.

Finally there is the moral/ethical issue. A judge may rule that the tax avoidance is legally effective and HMRC may not be able to prove it represents an artificial transaction. In this case the avoidance will work and the taxpayer will save tax but this doesn't make it right. Surely taxpayers should not be avoiding tax and a tax adviser should not be assisting them to do so?

Real life example

If you do an internet search for 'celebrity tax avoiders' you will find some interesting stories!

4.3 Tax evasion

This is illegal. This involves clearly breaking the tax law, for example failing to declare the profits of a business.

4.4 Summary

These distinctions are not always clear cut. It is best to see this as a spectrum, it is not always obvious where tax planning ends and mild tax avoidance begins or the point at which aggressive potentially illegal tax avoidance becomes illegal tax evasion.

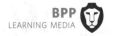

5 Professional conduct in relation to taxation

These are the rules that govern the relationship between a tax adviser and his client and HMRC.

The detailed rules are available to you in your assessment and are included in the *reference material and tax tables* at the back of this book. We recommend that you read these carefully. As they are available to you in the assessment you don't need to learn this information word for word but it is important that you remember the gist of it and know where to find the various sections.

To summarise, a tax practitioner should act in the best interests of their client, however, they must deal with HMRC staff in an open and constructive manner consistent with the law.

A tax adviser must follow the fundamental principles, particularly that of confidentiality.

A tax return may be prepared by an adviser but ultimately it is the taxpayer's responsibility and must be approved by the taxpayer before being submitted. The adviser should make this clear to the taxpayer and highlight any areas where they have had to exercise their judgement when preparing the return.

Providing tax advice is an ethically complex area for an adviser.

If a tax adviser learns of an error, omission or a failure to file a tax return, the adviser should bring this to the taxpayer's attention and request permission to disclose this to HMRC.

If the taxpayer refuses to disclose, then the adviser should notify the taxpayer in writing that they are unable to continue to act for them.

If the tax adviser works in an organisation they must report this to their Money Laundering Reporting Officer or, if the adviser is a sole practitioner directly to the National Crime Agency (NCA). The taxpayer should not be advised that a report has been made.

The adviser should consider whether to advise HMRC that previous information cannot be relied upon and consider how to answer any requests from a potential new adviser.

Usually, a practitioner would only disclose information to HMRC with the taxpayer's permission. In limited circumstances though, HMRC may gain access to information without the client's permission. This is a complex area.

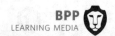

Activity 1: Irregularities

You act as tax adviser for Frank who is self-employed. Frank is currently divorcing his wife Vivien. You receive a large parcel from Vivien containing some significant sales invoices that Vivien says Frank has deliberately excluded from his accounting profits. **What action should you take?**

Solution

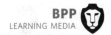

Chapter summary

- Governments collect taxation to raise finance, redistribute wealth, control the economy and encourage or discourage certain activities.

- Taxes should be neutral, efficient, simple, certain, effective and fair.

- The tax structure depends upon the tax base used and the tax rate applied.

- Individuals may have to pay income tax, capital gains tax, National Insurance and/or inheritance tax.

- Tax rates may be progressive, regressive or proportional.

- HMRC is responsible for the administration of tax.

- The tax year runs from 6 April in one year to the 5 April in the next year.

- Some of the rules governing tax are laid down in legislation, while some are laid down in case law.

- HMRC provides guidance about how tax law works.

- Residence and domicile are important concepts which determine how a taxpayer is taxed on UK and overseas income and assets.

- Tax evasion is illegal, tax planning is legal and tax avoidance may or may not be technically legal but is sometimes ethically wrong.

- Tax practitioners have responsibilities to their clients and to HMRC.

- The tax return is ultimately the client's responsibility.

- Providing tax advice is an ethically complex area.

- The ethical Guideline of confidentiality means that a client's tax affairs should not be discussed with third parties without the client's permission unless there is a legal right or obligation for the adviser to disclose the information.

- Tax practitioners may be required to produce information to HMRC.

- A tax practitioner must cease to act for a client who refuses to disclose an error or omission to HMRC, and must make a money laundering report.

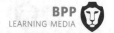

Keywords

- **Acts of Parliament:** laws produced by MPs debating in Parliament
- **Capital gains tax:** tax charged on the profits made on the disposal of capital items
- **Case law:** decisions of the Tax Tribunal about the interpretation of tax statutes which serve as a further source of tax law
- **Domicile:** a long-term test to identify whether the UK is a taxpayer's real home
- **Her Majesty's Revenue & Customs (HMRC):** responsible for the administration of tax
- **Income tax:** tax charged on money a taxpayer regularly receives
- **Inheritance tax:** tax charged on transfer of wealth
- **Legislation:** laws created by the Government. These include Acts of Parliament and Statutory Instruments
- **National Insurance:** tax paid on earnings from employment or self-employment
- **Progressive tax:** tax rate increases as the tax base increases
- **Proportional tax:** tax rate stays the same as the tax base changes
- **Regressive tax:** tax rate decreases as the tax base increases
- **Residence:** a short-term test to identify whether someone is present in the UK for tax purposes in a tax year
- **Statutory instrument:** laws produced by civil servants acting on behalf of the Chancellor of the Exchequer
- **Tax avoidance:** using the tax legislation in a way that was not intended to reduce tax liabilities. May or may not be technically illegal but sometimes ethically wrong.
- **Tax base:** the amount that will be taxed
- **Tax evasion:** breaking the law and not paying the correct amount of tax
- **Tax planning:** taking advantage of legal means by which a taxpayer may reduce their tax bill
- **Tax rate:** the percentage applied to the tax base
- **Tax structure:** the way the tax system has been organised
- **The tax year (fiscal year or year of assessment):** the 12-month period that runs from 6 April in one year to 5 April in the next year. Thus the tax year 2016/17 runs from 6 April 2016 to 5 April 2017

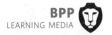

Activity 1: Irregularities

You should confirm the invoices are genuine and that they have been omitted from the accounts. You should then raise the matter with Frank and advise him that HMRC should be notified of the extra income, and that tax and potentially interest and penalties will be due.

If he agrees you should disclose the extra income to HMRC.

If he refuses you should advise him of the consequences first verbally and, if he still refuses, in writing. If he refuses to disclose the information you should cease to act for him and confirm this to him in writing.

You need to advise HMRC that you no longer act for him but you cannot say why as this would breach client confidentiality. You must consider making a money laundering report and consider whether you need to advise HMRC that any previous information supplied can no longer be relied on.

You need to consider carefully your response to any correspondence from a future adviser requesting whether Frank would be a suitable client.

Test your learning

1   **Identify whether the statement below is true or false.**

Statement	True ✓	False ✓
All taxpayers are sent a tax return each year by HM Revenue & Customs.		

2   The tax administration within the UK is undertaken by:

Tick ONE box.

	✓
The Chancellor of the Exchequer	
Companies House	
HM Revenue & Customs	
Members of Parliament	

3   **Indicate with ticks which TWO of the following have the force of law.**

	✓
Acts of Parliament	
HMRC Statements of practice	
Statutory Instruments	
Extra statutory concessions	

4   When is a tax practitioner not bound by the ethical guidelines of client confidentiality?

Tick ONE box.

	✓
When in a social environment	
When discussing client affairs with third parties with the client's proper and specific authority	
When reading documents relating to a client's affairs in public places	
When preparing tax returns	

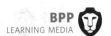
BPP
LEARNING MEDIA

5   Who should a sole practitioner make a report to if they suspect a client of money laundering?

Tick ONE box.

	✓
HMRC	
Nearest police station	
National Crime Agency	
Tax Tribunal	

6   Cornelius is an acquaintance of your client, Ruby, as they have similar jobs in similar sized companies. He knows that Ruby was made redundant recently. He is facing redundancy himself and would like to know how much redundancy money Ruby received so that he can compare this to the figure his company is offering him.

State how you should reply to his request for this information, clearly justifying your reply.

7   An ISA is a special bank account where cash may be saved and any interest earned is not subject to tax. David invests his redundancy money in an ISA. David is engaged in:

Tick ONE box.

	✓
Tax planning	
Tax avoidance	
Tax evasion	
Not possible to say until decided by a judge	

8   In country Z income tax is levied at a flat rate of 10% on all earnings. The tax rate is:

Tick ONE box.

	✓
Progressive	
Regressive	
Proportional	
Equitable	

9   James leaves the UK to work abroad for five years. He intends to return to the UK and stay there once the job ends. James's UK status is:

Tick ONE box.

	✓
Not resident or domiciled	
Not resident but domiciled	
Resident but not domiciled	
Resident and domiciled	

10 Pierre comes to visit the UK for the first time for a three-month period. He does not work in the UK during this period. He deposits money in a UK bank account and earns interest. He also receives rental income overseas and brings some of it into the UK. Pierre will be:

Tick ONE box.

	✓
Taxed on all of his income in the UK regardless as to where it is earned	
Taxed in the UK on his UK income and income brought into the UK from overseas	
Taxed in the UK only on his UK income	
Not taxed in the UK	

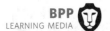

National Insurance

2

Learning outcomes

3	Calculate income tax and National Insurance (NI) contributions payable by a UK taxpayer
3.4	Calculate NI contributions for employees and employers
	• Identify taxpayers who need to pay NI
	• Calculate NI contributions payable by employees
	• Calculate NI contributions payable by employers

Assessment context

Task 7 in the initial AAT sample assessment tested the calculation of Class 1 Primary (employee), Class 1 Secondary (employer) and Class 1A (employer) National Insurance for 4 marks.

Qualification context

You will not see the information in this chapter outside of this unit.

Business context

National Insurance is a significant extra cost for an employer and an employee. An employer will have to consider the National Insurance cost when taking on new staff or offering increased salary or benefits to their existing staff.

Chapter overview

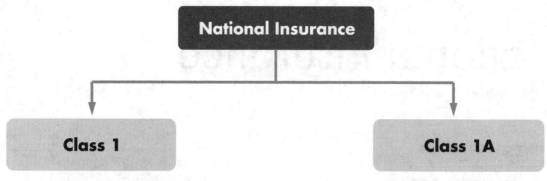

National Insurance

Class 1

- On cash earnings
- Exclude reimbursed expenses
- Include excessive mileage payments > 45p/mile
- Calculate weekly or monthly
- Annual calculation for directors

Class 1A

- Payable by employer
- On benefits
- Rate 13.8%

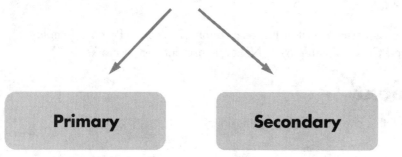

Primary

- Cost to employee
- £1 – £8,060   0 %
- £8,061 – £43,000 12%
- £43,001 and above 2%

Secondary

- Cost to employer
- £1 – £8,112   0%
- £8,113 and above 13.8%
- Deduct employment allowance of £3,000 from total bill

Introduction

An employer will have to deduct **Class 1 primary National Insurance** from their employees' cash earnings and pay this over to HMRC. This is a cost to the employee. In addition to this they will have to pay over **Class 1 secondary National Insurance** on the employees' cash earnings as well as **Class 1A National Insurance** on non-cash benefits received by the employee (for example use of a car owned by the company). Both of these represent an additional cost to the employer.

1 Class 1 Primary (Employee) National Insurance

Class 1 primary (Employee) National Insurance	This is deducted by the employer from the employees' earnings. It thus represents a cost to the employee.

1.1 What are earnings?

'Earnings' broadly comprise gross cash payments, excluding benefits which cannot be turned into cash by surrender (eg holidays). **Certain payments are exempt.** In general the income tax and NIC exemptions mirror one another so if a payment is exempt for income tax it is also exempt for National Insurance. We will consider exempt payments in detail in Chapter 4 but for example if an employee works away from home his employer can pay him up to £5 a night to cover incidental expenses and these payments would not be chargeable to income tax or National Insurance.

An expense with a business purpose is not treated as earnings. For example, if an employee is reimbursed for business travel or for staying in a hotel on the employer's business this is not normally 'earnings'

In general, vouchers are subject to Class 1 Primary and Secondary as they are deemed to be a cash equivalent. For exempt vouchers see Chapter 4.

1.2 Rates of contributions

The rates of contribution for 2016/17, and the income bands to which they apply, are provided in the assessment and set out in the *Reference material and tax tables* section at the end of this Course Book.

Employees pay Class 1 primary contributions at 12% of earnings between the primary threshold (PT) of £8,060 and the upper earnings limit (UEL) of £43,000 or the equivalent monthly or weekly limit (see below). They also pay additional Class 1 primary contributions of 2% on earnings above the upper earnings limit.

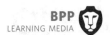

Illustration 1: Class 1 primary National Insurance

Sally works for Red plc. She is paid £4,000 per month. Show Sally's primary contributions deducted by Red plc for 2016/17.

Annual salary £4,000 × 12 = £48,000

Primary contributions	£
£(43,000 – 8,060) = £34,940 × 12% (main)	4,193
£(48,000 – 43,000) = £5,000 × 2% (additional)	100
Total primary contributions	4,293

Activity 1: Class 1 primary National Insurance

Tyrone is one of 3,000 employees of Taverner plc.

	£
Salary for 2016/17	45,000
Non cash benefits	6,450

What amount of national insurance does Tyrone suffer in the tax year?

£ [   ]

2 Class 1 secondary (Employer) National Insurance

Key term

Class 1 secondary (Employer) National Insurance	This is paid by the employer on top of the employees' earnings. It thus represents a cost to the employer.

2.1 What are earnings?

We use the same figure we calculated for the primary calculation above.

2.2 Rates of contributions

The rates of contribution for 2016/17, and the income bands to which they apply, are provided in the assessment and set out in the *Reference material and tax tables* section at the end of this Course Book.

Employers pay secondary contributions of 13.8% on earnings above the secondary threshold (ST) of £8,112, or the equivalent monthly or weekly limit. There is no upper limit.

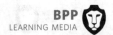

Illustration 2: Class 1 secondary National Insurance

Sally works for Red plc. She is paid £4,000 per month.

Show Sally's secondary contributions paid by Red plc for 2016/17.

Annual salary £4,000 × 12 = £48,000

Secondary threshold £8,112

Red plc	£
Secondary contributions	
£(48,000 – 8,112) = £39,888 × 13.8%	5,505

Activity 2: Class 1 secondary National Insurance

Tyrone is one of 3,000 employees of Taverner plc.

	£
Salary for 2016/17	45,000
Non cash benefits	6,450

What amount of Class 1 secondary national insurance does Tyrone's employer pay in the tax year? £ [   ]

3 Earnings periods for Class 1 primary and secondary National Insurance

In practice National Insurance is calculated with reference to the employee's earnings period so an employee who is paid weekly will have their National Insurance calculated using weekly thresholds and an employee who is paid monthly will have their National Insurance calculated using the monthly thresholds.

	Weekly £	Monthly £	Annual £
Primary Threshold (PT)	155	672	8,060
Secondary Threshold (ST)	156	676	8,112
Upper Earnings Limit (UEL)	827	3,583	43,000

If the employee earns the same amount every week/month then the annual calculation we have previously calculated will yield the same result as the calculation based on the actual earnings period. If the employee earns different amounts in different periods then the annual calculation shortcut will not always give the correct result.

In your assessment you will probably have to perform an annual calculation unless you are instructed to do otherwise.

Directors have a greater degree of control over how they are paid than most employees. There is therefore a risk that they could manipulate the way they are paid to minimise their liability. To prevent this, their National Insurance is always calculated on a cumulative basis. The detail of this calculation is outside the scope of your studies but effectively it will yield the same result as the annual calculation.

Illustration 3: Earning periods for directors and other employees

Bill and Ben work for Weed Ltd. Bill is a monthly paid employee. Ben who is a director of Weed Ltd, is also paid monthly. Each is paid an annual salary of £40,800 in 2016/17 and each also received a bonus of £3,000 in December 2016.

Show the primary and secondary contributions for both Bill and Ben, using a monthly earnings period for Bill. Ignore the employment allowance (see next section).

Bill

Primary threshold £8,060/12 = £672
Secondary threshold £8,112/12 = £676
Upper earnings limit £43,000/12 = £3,583
Regular monthly earnings £40,800/12 = £3,400

Primary contributions

	£
11 months	
£(3,400 – 672) = £2,728 × 12% × 11 (main only)	3,601
1 month (December)	
£(3,583 – 672) = £2,911 × 12% (main)	349
£(3,400 + 3,000 – 3,583) = £2,817 × 2% (additional)	56
Total primary contributions	4,006

BPP
LEARNING MEDIA

Secondary contributions

	£
11 months	
£(3,400 – 676) = £2,724 × 13.8% × 11	4,135
1 month (December)	
£(3,400 + 3,000 – 676) = £5,724 × 13.8%	790
Total secondary contributions	4,925

Ben

Total earnings £(40,800 + 3,000) = £43,800

Primary contributions

	£
Total earnings exceed UEL	
£(43,000 – 8,060) = £34,940 × 12% (main)	4,193
£(43,800 – 43,000) = £800 × 2% (additional)	16
Total primary	4,209

Secondary contributions

	£
£(43,800 – 8,112) = £35,688 × 13.8%	4,925

Because Ben is a director an annual earnings period applies. The effect of this is that increased primary contributions are due.

4 The employment allowance

An employer can make a claim to **reduce its total Class 1 secondary contributions** by an **employment allowance equal to those contributions**, subject to a **maximum allowance of £3,000 per tax year**.

Some employers are **excluded employers** for the purposes of the employment allowance. These include those who employ **employees for personal, household or domestic work, public authorities** and employers who **carry out functions either wholly or mainly of a public nature** such as provision of National Health Service services. Companies where the director is the only employee are also excluded from the employment allowance from 2016/17.

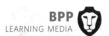

Illustration 4: The employment allowance

Blue plc is a trading company which has two employees, one who earns £20,000 per year and the other who earns £30,000 per year. Each employee is paid in equal monthly amounts and so an annual computation of Class 1 computation can be made.

Calculate the Class 1 secondary contributions payable by Blue plc for 2016/17.

	£
Employee 1: £(20,000 – 8,112) = 11,888 × 13.8%	1,641
Employee 2: £(30,000 – 8,112) = 21,888 × 13.8%	3,021
	4,662
Less employment allowance (maximum)	(3,000)
Secondary contributions 2016/17	1,662

Activity 3: The employment allowance

Stoney Heap Ltd is a trading company which has two employees, one earns £18,000 per year and the other earns £15,000 per year. Each employee is paid in equal monthly amounts.

How much Class 1 secondary contributions are payable by Stoney Heap Ltd for 2016/17? £ [ ]

5 Class 1A National Insurance

Key term

Class 1A National Insurance	This is paid by the employer on the cash value of employees' non cash benefits. It is paid in addition to the benefits. It thus represents a cost to the employer.

5.1 What are benefits?

If an employee is provided with non-cash benefits such as the use of a car belonging to the employer then we must calculate a cash equivalent value so that income tax and National Insurance may be applied. The calculation of the cash equivalent value is addressed in Chapter 4.

Assessment focus point

In National Insurance questions you will probably be given the value of the benefit although you may be expected to apply the rules in Chapter 4 to calculate it.

5.2 Rates of contributions

The rates of contribution for 2016/17, and the income bands to which they apply, are provided in the assessment and set out in the *Reference material and tax tables* section of this Course Book.

We simply apply 13.8% to the cash value of the benefits.

Illustration 5: Class 1A National Insurance

Sally has the following benefits for income tax purposes

	£
Company car	5,200
Living accommodation	10,000
Medical insurance	800

Calculate the Class 1A NICs that the employer will have to pay.

Total benefits are £16,000 (£10,000 + £5,200 + £800)

Class 1A NICs:

£16,000 × 13.8% = £2,208

Activity 4: Class 1A National Insurance

Tyrone is one of 3,000 employees of Taverner plc.

	£
Salary for 2016/17	45,000
Non-cash benefits	6,450

The Class 1A National Insurance payable by Taverner plc is

£ [   ]

6 Reimbursed expenses including business mileage

As noted above, reimbursement of genuine expenses incurred in doing your job are not subject to class 1 National Insurance.

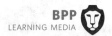

However, if the employer was paying for a private expense of the employee it would be subject to National Insurance. For example if the employer reimbursed the employee for specific business phone calls National Insurance would not apply. If the employer paid for all of the employee's calls class 1 primary and secondary would be applied to the cost of the private calls reimbursed.

An employee may use his own car on his employer's business and be reimbursed for the cost he has incurred. The employer may reimburse up to 45p a mile without any National Insurance implications. Any sums paid in excess of 45p would be subject to Class 1 primary and secondary National Insurance. Note this is slightly different to the income tax treatment we will see in Chapter 4 where a lower rate applies after 10,000 miles have been driven in a tax year.

Illustration 6: Business mileage

Sophie uses her own car for business travel. During 2016/17, Sophie drove 15,400 miles in the performance of her duties. Sophie's employer paid her a mileage allowance. How is the mileage allowance treated for National Insurance purposes assuming that the rate paid is:

(a) 40p a mile?
(b) 50p a mile?

(a)

	£
Mileage allowance received (15,400 × 40p)	6,160
Permitted payment (15,400 × 45p)	(6,930)
Excess over limit	0

As the payment is within the permitted amount there is no charge to National Insurance

(b)

	£
Mileage allowance received (15,400 × 50p)	7,700
Less tax free amount (above)	(6,930)
	770

As the payment is above the permitted amount the excess of £770 will be chargeable to Class 1 National Insurance, primary and secondary

7 Tax planning

An employee may choose to receive non-cash benefits rather than a cash pay rise as cash earnings would be subject to Class 1 primary whereas benefits would not be. The employer would probably be indifferent here between providing cash and benefits as cash would be subject to Class 1 secondary whereas benefits would be subject to Class 1A, both at 13.8%.

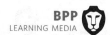

Chapter summary

- Class 1 National Insurance is applied to an employee's cash earnings from employment. Vouchers are included but reimbursed business expenses are excluded.

- Class 1 primary is deducted from an employee's earnings. It is therefore a cost to the employee.

- Class 1 secondary is paid in addition to an employee's earnings. It is therefore a cost to the employer.

- Class 1 primary and secondary are usually calculated with reference to an employee's earnings period, weekly or monthly. If the employee earns the same amount each period an annual shortcut calculation can be done instead.

- Directors will have their NIC calculated on a cumulative basis meaning that the annual calculation will always give the correct result.

- An employer is allowed to deduct the employment allowance from the Class 1 secondary liability reducing the cost to them.

- Class 1A is payable by the employer on the cash equivalent value of non-cash benefits received by the employee.

- There is no Class 1 on the reimbursement of genuine business expenses but if the employer pays a private expense of the employee it will be subject to National Insurance. This includes excessive payments to an employee for the use of their own car.

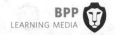

Keywords

- **Class 1 primary National Insurance (employee):** the National Insurance deducted from an employee's earnings

- **Class 1 secondary National Insurance (employer):** the National Insurance an employer pays on top of an employee's earnings

- **Class 1A National Insurance (employer):** the National Insurance an employer pays on the value of non-cash benefits received by an employee

- **Employment allowance:** an amount that can be deducted from the employer's Class 1 secondary liability

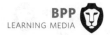

Activity 1: Class 1 primary National Insurance

The class 1 primary National Insurance is £ | 4,233 |

Workings:

Tyrone suffers Class 1 primary contributions on his cash earnings.

Class 1 primary

$(43,000 - 8,060) \times 12\% =$ 4,193

$(45,000 - 43,000) \times 2\% =$ <u>40</u>

                     <u>4,233</u>

Activity 2: Class 1 secondary National Insurance

The class 1 secondary National Insurance is £ | 5,091 |

Workings:

Class 1 secondary

$(45,000 - 8,112) \times 13.8\% =$ <u>5,091</u>

Activity 3: The employment allowance

The class 1 secondary National Insurance is £ | 0 |

Workings

	£
Employee 1: £(18,000 – 8,112) × 13.8%	1,365
Employee 2: £(15,000 – 8,112) × 13.8%	951
	2,316
Less employment allowance (maximum £3,000, restricted)	(2,316)
Secondary contributions	0

Activity 4: Class 1A National Insurance

The Class 1A National Insurance payable by Taverner plc is £ | 890 |

Workings:

Class 1A

6,450 @ 13.8% =   <u>890</u>

Test your learning

1 Robert is one of 3,000 employees of George plc. He receives the following from his employer in tax year 2016/17:

	£
Salary	42,000
Reimbursed business expenses	3,000
Non cash benefits	8,000

What amount of Class 1 primary National Insurance contributions does Robert's employer pay over on his behalf? £ [ ]

What amount of secondary National Insurance contributions does Robert's employer pay in the tax year? £ [ ]

What amount of class 1A National Insurance contributions does Robert's employer pay in the tax year? £ [ ]

2 Alec works for Knight Ltd. He is paid monthly and receives an annual salary of £36,000 in 2016/17. He also receives a bonus of £10,000 in March 2017.

Show the primary and secondary contributions for Alec using a monthly earnings period. Ignore the employment allowance.

Alec's primary contributions are £ [ ]

Alec's secondary contributions are £ [ ]

3 Elizabeth is a director of Faerie plc. She is paid monthly and receives an annual salary of £36,000 in 2016/17 and receives a bonus of £10,000 in March 2017.

Show the primary and secondary contributions for Elizabeth. Ignore the employment allowance.

Elizabeth's primary contributions are £ [ ]

Elizabeth's secondary contributions are £ [ ]

4 Ursa Minor Beta plc is a trading company which has two employees, one earns £25,000 per year and the other who earns £60,000 per year. Each employee is paid in equal monthly amounts.

The Class 1 secondary contributions payable by Ursa Minor Beta Ltd are £ [ ]

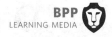

5   Toby uses his own car for business travel. During 2016/17, Toby drove 18,500 miles in the performance of his duties. Toby's employer paid him a mileage allowance.

If the mileage allowance is 35p a mile the amount subject to Class 1 National Insurance is £ [   ]

If the mileage allowance is 50p a mile the amount subject to Class 1 National Insurance is £ [   ]

Inheritance tax

3

Learning outcomes

1	Analyse the theories, principles and rules that underpin taxation systems
1.4	**Discuss residence and domicile** • The definitions of residence and domicile • The impact that each of these has on the taxation position of a UK taxpayer
5	**Discuss the basics of inheritance tax**
5.1	**Identify the basic features of chargeable lifetime and exempt transfers** • Chargeable lifetime transfers • Exempt transfers • Potential exempt transfers
5.2	**Perform basic inheritance tax computations** • Calculate tax payable on death • Calculate tax payable on lifetime transfers • Identify who is responsible for payment of inheritance tax

Assessment context

Inheritance tax is worth 12% of the total syllabus so in your assessment you should expect to see questions worth approximately 12% of the total marks available.

In the initial sample assessment released by the AAT, Task 12 tested various inheritance tax rules for 6 marks while Task 13 required you to input a detailed inheritance tax calculation into a free text box.

Qualification context

You will not see the information in this chapter outside of this unit.

Business context

A tax practitioner may have to advise a taxpayer how to structure their tax affairs during lifetime to minimise the tax liability on their death. A practitioner may have to perform lifetime inheritance tax calculations for their clients and produce inheritance tax calculations on behalf of the executors of clients who have died.

Chapter overview

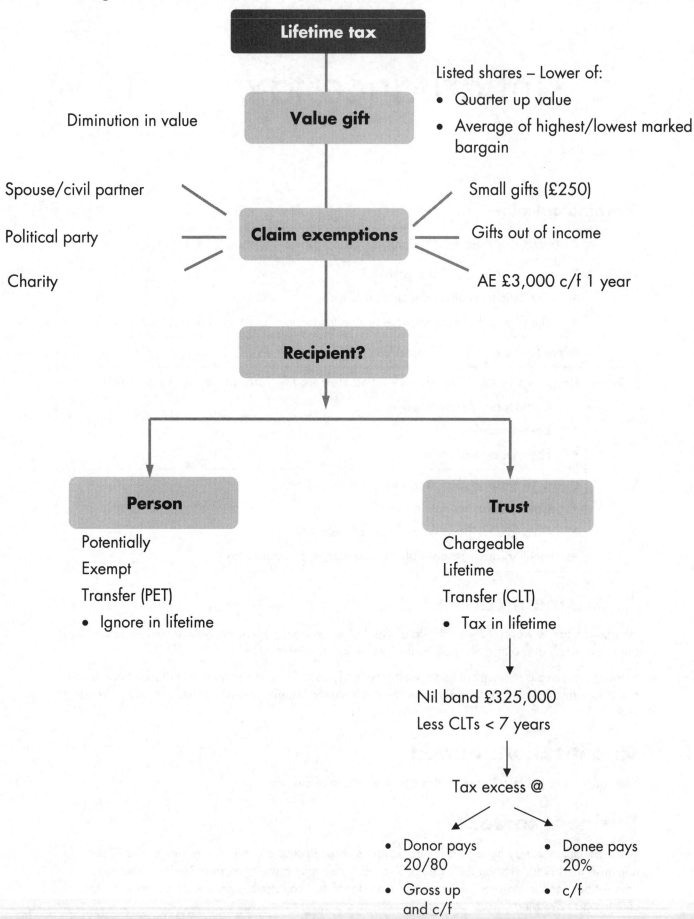

Lifetime tax

Value gift

Diminution in value

Listed shares – Lower of:
- Quarter up value
- Average of highest/lowest marked bargain

Claim exemptions

Spouse/civil partner

Political party

Charity

Small gifts (£250)

Gifts out of income

AE £3,000 c/f 1 year

Recipient?

Person

Potentially
Exempt
Transfer (PET)
- Ignore in lifetime

Trust

Chargeable
Lifetime
Transfer (CLT)
- Tax in lifetime

Nil band £325,000
Less CLTs < 7 years

Tax excess @

- Donor pays 20/80
- Gross up and c/f

- Donee pays 20%
- c/f

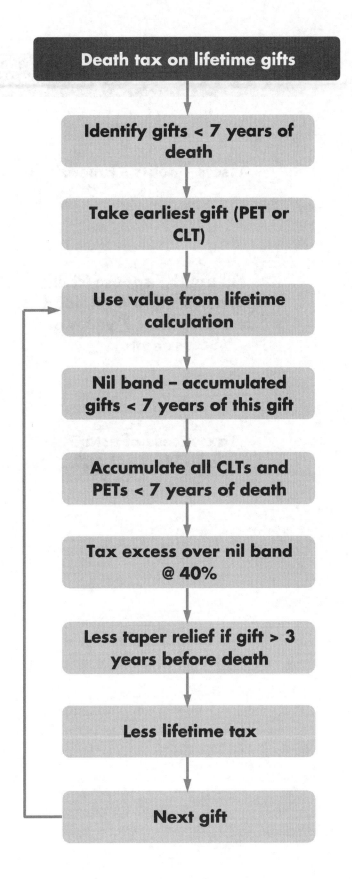

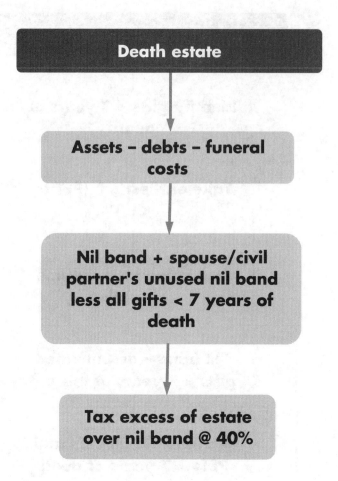

Introduction

Key term

Inheritance tax	This is a tax on the transfer of wealth
	Only individuals pay inheritance tax. It is not levied on companies or partnerships.
	Don't make the mistake of thinking inheritance tax is only applicable on death, it can also apply to transfers of wealth made during lifetime.
Transfer of wealth	This is when a taxpayer deliberately gives away their wealth and receives either nothing in return or fails to obtain full value from the recipient. Inheritance tax therefore catches gifts or deliberate sales at undervalue.

Note that there has to be a **gratuitous intent** here, the taxpayer must have intended to give away their wealth. There is therefore no inheritance tax charge if a tax payer simply makes a bad bargain, for example selling a painting for £500 that turns out to be worth £5,000.

Questions will therefore talk about 'transfers' or 'gifts'.

To calculate inheritance tax it is important to realise it is a three stage process. All the three stages have to be calculated in the correct order as the first stage will have an impact on the second and the second on the third.

The three stages are:

- Lifetime tax paid on lifetime transfers
- Death tax paid on lifetime transfers made in the seven years prior to death
- Death tax paid on assets owned at death (death estate)

1 Domicile issues

Domicile is the key issue for inheritance tax (we covered the definition of domicile in Chapter 1).

If a taxpayer is UK domiciled they will be chargeable to inheritance tax on all the assets they own regardless of the location of the assets.

If a taxpayer is not UK domiciled they will be only taxed on assets located within the UK.

We will now consider the three stages in the computation. The first is the lifetime tax paid on lifetime transfers.

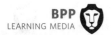

2 Lifetime tax paid on lifetime transfers

This is when a taxpayer makes a gift during life time which is subject to inheritance tax.

Donor	The person making a gift
Donee	The person receiving the gift

Key term

Tax is calculated with reference to the tax year.

The first step is always to value the gift.

2.1 Value of the transfer

The value of the transfer is calculated using the **diminution in value** principle.

In many cases the diminution in value of the donor's estate will be the same as the increase in the value of the donee's estate, for example if there is a cash gift or the gift of a house. However, sometimes the two will not be the same. Typically this is the situation where unquoted shares are gifted.

The measure of the transfer for inheritance tax purposes is always the loss to the donor (the diminution in value of his estate), not the amount gained by the donee.

Illustration 1: Diminution in value

Audrey wishes to give 200 shares to her son, Brian. Whilst the shares are only worth £2.50 each to Brian, since Brian will have only a small minority holding in the company, they were worth £15 each to Audrey as they gave her control of the company. After the gift Audrey will hold 4,900 shares and the value of these shares will be £10 each. The value per share to Audrey falls from £15 to £10 per share since she will lose control of the company.

The diminution in value of Audrey's estate is £27,500, as follows.

	£
Before the gift: 5,100 shares × £15	76,500
After the gift: 4,900 shares × £10	(49,000)
Diminution in value	27,500

Activity 1: Diminution of value

Mr Jones owns 75% of Hill Jones Ltd, an unquoted investment company. He gives a 30% holding to his son.

Shareholdings on this date were valued at:

Shareholding	£
75%	370,000
45%	200,000
30%	105,000

What is the value of the gift for inheritance tax purposes?

£ [   ]

2.2 Listed shares

Note there are special rules that apply when the gift is of listed shares.

Quoted shares and securities are valued at the lower of:

- The 'quarter up' value: lower quoted price plus ¼ (higher quoted price – lower quoted price)

- The average of the highest and lowest marked bargains

Illustration 2: Valuing listed shares

Shares in A plc are given away. On the day of the disposal they are quoted at 100–110p. The highest and lowest marked bargains were 99p and 110p.

The value per share is the lower of:

(a) 100 + ¼ (110 – 100) = 102.5p
(b) 110 + 99/2 = 104.5p

The value per share is 102.5p

2.3 Exemptions

Once we have valued the gift we then need to consider whether it is eligible for exemptions.

Some exemptions are only available on lifetime gifts while others are available on both lifetime and death gifts.

There are far more exemptions available during lifetime than on death so from a tax planning perspective it usually makes sense to give assets away during lifetime and use the exemptions to reduce the tax bill rather than allowing them to pass on your death when it is likely that more tax will have to be paid.

2.3.1 Exemptions that are always available during lifetime and on death

2.3.1.1 Transfers between spouses/civil partners

Any transfers of value between spouses/civil partners are exempt. The exemption covers lifetime gifts between them and property passing under a will or on intestacy. Intestacy is when the taxpayer has not made a will so their assets pass on to relatives following rules created by the government.

2.3.1.2 Transfers to charities/political parties

These are always exempt.

2.3.2 Exemptions only available during lifetime

2.3.2.1 The small gifts exemptions

Outright gifts to individuals totalling £250 or less per donee in any one tax year are exempt. If gifts total more than £250 the whole amount is chargeable. A donor can give up to £250 each year to each of as many donees as he wishes. The small gifts exemption cannot apply to gifts into trusts. We will discuss trusts later.

2.3.2.2 The annual exemption (AE)

The first £3,000 of value transferred in a tax year is exempt from IHT. The annual exemption is used only after all other exemptions (such as for transfers to spouses/civil partners). If several gifts are made in a year, the £3,000 exemption is applied to earlier gifts before later gifts.

Any unused portion of the annual exemption is carried forward for one year only. Only use it the following year after that year's annual exemption has been used.

Illustration 3: Annual exempt amount

Frank has no unused annual exemption brought forward at 6 April 2015.

On 1 August 2015 he makes a transfer of £600 to his son Peter.

On 1 September 2015 he makes a transfer of £2,000 to his nephew Quentin.

On 1 July 2016 he makes a transfer of £3,300 to a trust for his grandchildren.

On 1 June 2017 he makes a transfer of £5,000 to his friend Rowan.

Show the application of the annual exemptions.

2015/16	£
1.8.15 Gift to Peter	600
Less AE 2015/16	(600)
	0

	£
1.9.15 Gift to Quentin	2,000
Less AE 2015/16	(2,000)
	0

The unused annual exemption carried forward is £3,000 – £600 – £2,000 = £400.

2016/17	£	£
1.7.16 Gift to trust		3,300
Less: AE 2016/17	3,000	
AE 2015/16 b/f	300	
		(3,300)
		0

The unused annual exemption carried forward is zero because the 2016/17 exemption must be used before the 2015/16 exemption brought forward. The balance of £100 of the 2015/16 exemption is lost, because it cannot be carried forward for more than one year.

2017/18	£
1.6.17 Gift to Rowan	5,000
Less AE 2017/18	(3,000)
	2,000

2.3.2.3 Normal expenditure out of income

Inheritance tax is a tax on transfers of capital, not income. A transfer of value is exempt if:

(a) It is made as part of the normal expenditure of the donor

(b) Taking one year with another, it was made out of income

(c) It leaves the donor with sufficient income to maintain his usual standard of living

As well as covering such things as regular presents this exemption can cover regular payments out of income such as a grandchild's school fees or the payment of life assurance premiums on a policy for someone else.

2.3.2.4 Gifts in consideration of marriage/civil partnership

Gifts in consideration of marriage/civil partnership are exempt up to:

(a)   £5,000 if from a parent of a party to the marriage/civil partnership

(b)   £2,500 if from a remoter ancestor or from one of the parties to the marriage/civil partnership

(c)   £1,000 if from any other person

The limits apply to gifts from any one donor for any one marriage/civil partnership. The exemption is available only if the marriage/civil partnership actually takes place. This exemption is deducted before the annual exemption.

Assessment focus point

These exemptions are given to you in the assessment.

Illustration 4: Exemptions

Dale made a gift of £153,000 to her son on 17 October 2012 on the son's marriage. Dale gave £100,000 to her spouse on 1 January 2016. Dale gave £70,000 to her daughter on 11 May 2016. The only other gifts Dale made were birthday and Christmas presents of £100 each to her grandchildren.

The following exemptions are available in respect of these transfers:

17 October 2012

	£
Gift to Dale's son	153,000
Less: ME	(5,000)
AE 2012/13	(3,000)
AE 2011/12 b/f	(3,000)
	142,000

1 January 2016

	£
Gift to Dale's spouse	100,000
Less spouse exemption	(100,000)
	0

11 May 2016

	£
Gift to Dale's daughter	70,000
Less: AE 2016/17	(3,000)
AE 2015/16 b/f	(3,000)
	64,000

The gifts to the grandchildren are covered by the small gifts exemption.

2.4 Is the gift taxable during lifetime?

Once we have valued the gift and deducted any exemptions we now need to consider whether it is actually taxable during lifetime.

A lifetime gift can be one of two things:

Key term

Potentially Exempt Transfer (PET)	This is a gift to an individual. It is not taxable during lifetime but will be charged to inheritance tax if the donor dies within seven years of making the gift.
Chargeable Lifetime Transfer (CLT)	This is a gift to a trust. It is immediately chargeable to inheritance tax during lifetime and will be charged to tax a second time if the donor dies within seven years of making the gift.

A trust arises when the law recognises that one party (the trustee(s)) is/are looking after an asset on behalf of another person/people (the beneficiary/beneficiaries).

Note that although PETs are not chargeable during lifetime is important to consider them as they will use annual exemptions that could have been used by CLTs and if the taxpayer dies within seven years of making the PET we will have to tax them.

There is an important tax planning point here. When CLTs and PETS are made in the same year the CLTs should be made first to use any available annual exemptions. If used up against the PETs the exemption(s) will be wasted if the donor survives seven years as the PET then will never be chargeable.

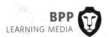

2.5 Calculation of lifetime tax on CLTs

Lifetime inheritance tax on lifetime transfers is chargeable at two rates of tax: a 0% rate (the 'nil rate') and 20%. The nil rate is chargeable where accumulated transfers do not exceed the nil rate band limit. The excess is chargeable at 20%.

The nil rate band is £325,000.

Accumulated transfers	These are CLTs made in the previous seven years.

Key term

2.5.1 Donee pays the tax

When a CLT is made and the donee (ie the trustee) pays the lifetime tax, follow these steps to work out the lifetime inheritance tax on it:

Step 1

Compute the value of the CLT. You may be given this in the question or you may have to work out the diminution of value or use the listed shares rules. You would then deduct exemptions (such as the annual exemption).

Step 2

Look back seven years from the date of the transfer to see if any other CLTs have been made. If so, these transfers use up the nil rate band available for the current transfer. This is called seven year accumulation. Work out the value of any nil rate band still available.

Step 3

Any part of the CLT covered by the nil rate band is taxed at 0%. Any part of the CLT not covered by the nil rate band is charged at 20%.

Illustration 5: Tax payable by trustees

Eric makes a gift of £336,000 to a trust on 10 July 2016. The trustees agree to pay the tax due.

Calculate the lifetime tax payable by the trustees if Eric has made a lifetime chargeable transfer of value of £100,000 in August 2009.

Step 1

Value of CLT after exemptions (2 x £3,000) is £330,000.

Step 2

Lifetime transfer of value of £100,000 in seven years before 10 July 2016 (transfers after 10 July 2009). Nil rate band of £(325,000 – 100,000) £225,000 is available.

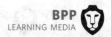

Step 3

	IHT £
£225,000 × 0%	0
£105,000 × 20%	21,000
£330,000	21,000

IHT due of £21,000

2.5.2 Donor pays the tax

Consider the situation where the donor has already made gifts over the nil rate band of £325,000. Any further gifts made will be subject to inheritance tax at 20%.

Imagine the donor wants the trust to have an additional £100,000. If the donor gives the trust £100,000 the trustee will have to account for tax at 20%. The trustee pays £20,000 leaving £80,000 in the trust. The trust now does not have the full amount the donor wanted it to have!

To get round this problem the donor may give the trust the amount he wanted the trust to have and then pay an additional sum to cover the tax payable on this amount. This is known as **grossing up** the gift.

The gross amount (gift + tax) represents 100%, the tax 20% and the amount after tax has been paid (**the net**) represents 80%. So if the donor wants the trust to have £100,000 and this represents 80%, the tax payable would be £100,000 × 20/80 = £25,000 and the gross amount £125,000 (£100,000 + £25,000). We can check this. If the donor pays £125,000 the tax is 20% of this, £25,000 leaving £100,000 for the trust.

It is normally assumed that the donor will pay the tax so the applicable rate is 20/80 which can be simplified to 25% or 1/4.

Assessment focus point

Read the question carefully to identify who is paying the tax. If the question is silent assume it is the donor who is paying the tax and use the 20/80 rate.

Note that a gift made now will impact on later gifts and may be taxed again if the donor dies within seven years of making the gift. It is important to therefore identify the value of the gift carried forward. If the donor pays the tax the loss to the donor is not the net gift but the gross amount as they have paid tax on top of the amount received by the trust. It is therefore the gross amount that is carried forward.

If the donor is paying the tax then our steps are slightly different.

Step 1

Compute the value of the gift. You may be given this in the question or you may have to work it out.

Step 2

Look back seven years from the date of the transfer to see if any other CLTs have been made. If so, these transfers use up the nil rate band available for the current transfer. Work out the value of any nil rate band still available.

Step 3

Any part of the CLT covered by the nil rate band is taxed at 0%. Any part of the CLT not covered by the nil rate band is taxed at 20/80.

Step 4

Work out the gross transfer by adding the net transfer and the tax together. You can check your figure by working out the tax on the gross transfer.

Illustration 6: Tax payable by donor

James makes a gift of £336,000 to a trust on 10 July 2016. James will pay the tax due.

Calculate the lifetime tax payable, if James has made a lifetime chargeable transfer of value of £100,000 in August 2009.

Step 1

Value of gift after exemptions (2 × £3,000) is £330,000.

Step 2

Lifetime transfer of value of £100,000 in seven years before 10 July 2016 (transfers after 10 July 2009). Nil rate band of £(325,000 – 100,000) = £225,000 available.

Step 3

	IHT £
£225,000 × 0%	0
£105,000 × 20/80	26,250
£330,000	26,250

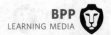

Step 4

Gross transfer is £(330,000 + 26,250) = £356,250.

Check: Tax on the gross transfer would be:

	IHT £
£225,000 × 0%	0
£131,250 × 20	26,250
£356,250	26,250

2.6 Lifetime tax summary

- Value gift

    - Diminution in value

- Deduct reliefs and exemptions

    - Marriage exemption
    - A/E(s)
    - Small gifts

- Is the gift a CLT or PET?

    - PET – ignore in lifetime
    - CLT – tax it!

- Deduct available nil band – £325,000 for 2016/17 less any CLTs in the previous seven years.

- Tax excess at 25% (20/80) if donor pays or 20% if trust pays. (If question is silent assume donor pays it).

- Gross value of gift (gross chargeable transfers (GCT).

    = gift (after all reliefs and exemptions) plus tax if donor pays
    = just gift (after all reliefs and exemptions) if trust pays

Illustration 7: Lifetime tax pro forma

		£
Lifetime tax:		
Gift		X
Less AE		(X)
Less AE b/f		(X)
Net gift after exemptions		X
Less: Nil band remaining:		
Nil band at date of gift	X	
Less: GCT's in last 7 years before gift	(X)	
		(X)
		X
Tax @ 20% (or $^{20}/_{80}$)		X

The gross chargeable transfer (GCT) which will use up the nil band for future gifts is calculated as follows:

		£
Net gift after exemptions		X
Tax paid by donor at $^{20}/_{80}$		X
		GCT

Activity 2: Calculating lifetime tax – CLTs only

Mr Butcher put £337,000 into a trust on 13 August 2016 having already put £116,000 into a trust three years earlier, (the gross chargeable transfer was £110,000).

Calculate the IHT payable when the trust is set up on 13 August 2016 and the gross chargeable transfer carried forward assuming:

(a)   The trust agrees to pay the tax

The tax payable is £ [   ]

The gross chargeable transfer is £ [   ]

(b)   Mr Butcher pays the tax.

The tax payable is £ [   ]

The gross chargeable transfer is £ [   ]

Activity 3: Calculating lifetime tax – PETs and CLTs

Mr Beale put £343,000 into a trust on 13 August 2016 (trustees agreeing to pay the tax) having given £50,000 to his daughter on 15 March 2016. He gave £30,000 to his son on 19 August 2016.

Calculate how much inheritance tax is payable on the:

(i)   Gift to daughter

The tax is £ [   ]

(ii)   Gift to trust

The tax is £ [   ]

(iii) Gift to son

The tax is £ [   ]

3 Death tax paid on lifetime transfers made in the seven years prior to death

Having considered the inheritance tax paid during lifetime the next step is to calculate inheritance tax payable on gifts made in the seven years prior to death.

Inheritance tax is charged on both PETs and CLTs made in the seven years prior to death.

It is important to note that gifts made more than seven years prior to the date of death will escape being charged to death tax. If the gift was a PET it would not have been taxed in lifetime either so we can now say it is no longer **potentially** exempt, it **is** exempt.

Note also that if a taxpayer survives more than three years after making the gift then the tax payable will be reduced by **taper relief**.

It is therefore an important tax planning point that wealth should be given away as soon as possible. If the donor survives seven years after making the gift there will be no death tax, if the donor survives at least three years there will be death tax but this will be reduced by taper relief. The longer the taxpayer waits before making the gift the less likely it is they will survive long enough to escape/reduce death tax.

Note that the death tax is always paid by the recipient of the gift.

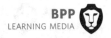

Follow these steps to work out the death tax on the lifetime gifts.

Step 1

Identify the date of death. Look back seven years and identify all lifetime transfers made in this period. These are now **chargeable** regardless as to whether they were made to a person or a trust.

Step 2

Start with the earliest gift made in the seven years prior to death:

- Establish the gross chargeable amount (this would have been done for CLT's in the lifetime calculation above ie value it, deduct exemptions, gross up for lifetime tax if necessary)

- Take the nil rate band at death and look back seven years from the date of the gift to see if there are any earlier gifts that will reduce the amount of nil rate band. Note that CLTs made more than seven years prior to the date of death will reduce the available nil rate band but PETs made more than seven years prior to death are now exempt so can be ignored.

- Deduct the remaining nil band from the gift under consideration and tax any excess at the **death rate** of 40%.

- Taper the tax if the gift was made more than three years before the date of death.

- Deduct any lifetime tax paid. The death tax can be reduced to nil but a tax refund cannot be generated.

Step 3

Repeat Step 2 for the next gift made in the seven year period prior to death. Note that when considering whether any of the nil band remains CLTs will always reduce the nil band regardless of when they were made but PETs will only reduce the nil band if made within seven years prior to the date of death.

Step 4

Repeat Step 2 for the next gift. Repeat for each of the gifts made in the seven years prior to death.

The taper relief rates are as follows:

Years before death	% reduction
Over three but less than four years	20
Over four but less than five years	40
Over five but less than six years	60
Over six but less than seven years	80

Illustration 8: Death tax on lifetime gifts

Boris Kartovski dies on 15 September 2016. You establish he has made the following gifts during his lifetime:

24 July 2005 CLT – gross chargeable transfer £300,000, no life time tax

1 August 2009 – PET – value after exemptions £500,000

13 January 2011 PET – value after exemptions £100,000

23 July 2013 CLT – gross chargeable transfer £400,000, life time tax £15,000

(At the date of this gift during lifetime the full nil band would have been available as the only gifts in the previous seven years were PETs. The donee paid the tax – (£400,000 – £325,000) × 20% = £15,000. As the donee paid the tax there is no need to gross up the gift.)

Refer to the following diagram as we work through the illustration.

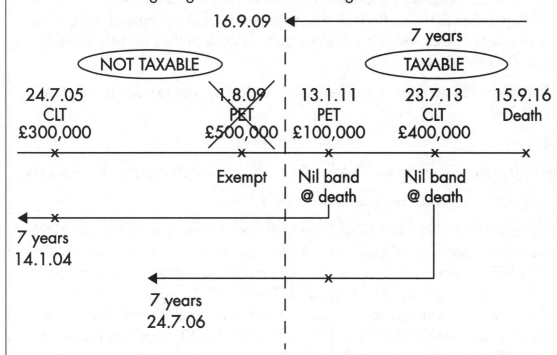

Step 1

Boris dies on 15 September 2016. All gifts made in the previous seven years are taxable regardless as to whether they were CLTs or PETs during lifetime. We are therefore interested in gifts made in the period 16 September 2009 to 15 September 2016.

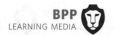

Step 2

The earliest gift made in the seven years prior to death is the PET made on 13 January 2011. This is now chargeable to death tax.

- The gross chargeable amount is £100,000

- The nil rate band at death is £325,000. If we look back seven years from 13 January 2011 to 14 January 2004 we see two earlier gifts made on the 24 July 2005 and 1 August 2009. One of these is a PET made more than seven years prior to the date of death so we can ignore it. The other though is a CLT so it will reduce our nil band. The nil band is therefore £325,000 – £300,000 = £25,000.

- The death tax on the gift is therefore (£100,000 – £25,000) × 40% = £30,000

- The gift was made on 13 January 2011 and death occurred on 15 September 2016 so Boris survived five years after the date of the gift but not six years. Taper relief is therefore 60% so 40% of the tax is chargeable £30,000 × 40% = £12,000

- This was a PET so there is no lifetime tax to deduct. The tax due is therefore £12,000.

Step 3

The next gift is the CLT made on 23 July 2013. This is now chargeable to death tax.

- The gross chargeable amount is £400,000

- The nil rate band is £325,000. If we look back seven years to 24 July 2006 we see two earlier gifts made on 1 August 2009 and 13 January 2011. Both were PETs in lifetime. The earlier PET was made more than seven years prior to the date of death so can be ignored. The later PET though has become chargeable to death tax so must be included in our calculation. The nil rate band is therefore £325,000 - £100,000 = £225,000. Note that the earlier CLT of £300,000 made on 24 July 2005 is now out of range.

- The death tax on the gift is therefore (£400,000 – £225,000) × 40% = £70,000.

- The gift was made on 23 July 2013 and death occurred on 15 September 2016 so Boris survived three years after the date of the gift but not four years. Taper relief is therefore 20% so 80% of the tax is chargeable £70,000 × 80% = £56,000

- This was a CLT so there is lifetime tax to deduct. The tax due is therefore £56,000 – £15,000 = £41,000.

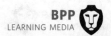

Illustration 9: Death tax on lifetime gifts pro forma

Death tax

	£	£
Gross CLT/PET		X
Less nil band remaining: Nil band on death	325,000	
Less GCTs in 7 years before **gift**	(X)	
Nil band remaining		(X)
		X
Tax @ 40%		IHT
Less taper relief		
% × IHT		(X)
		X
Less lifetime tax (on CLT)		(X)
Death tax due		X

Activity 4: Death tax on lifetime gifts 1

Mr Fowler made the following gifts during his lifetime:

3 March 2009	Gift to nephew	£40,000
14 October 2013	Gift to granddaughter on her marriage	£158,000
23 November 2014	Gift to son	£210,000

He died on 13 September 2016.

State the death tax payable on each of the gifts and who it is paid by:

(i) Gift to nephew

The tax is £ ☐

The tax is paid by ☐ ▼

Picklist:

Mr. Fowler
Nephew
nobody

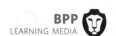

(ii) Gift to granddaughter

The tax is £ [   ]

The tax is paid by [▼]

Picklist:

granddaughter
Mr. Fowler's estate
nobody

(iii) Gift to son

The tax is £ [   ]

The tax is paid by [▼]

Picklist:

Mr. Fowler's estate
nobody
son

Activity 5: Death tax on lifetime gifts 2

Mr Raymond made the following gifts during his lifetime:

| 13 May 2011 | Gift to daughter | £130,000 |
| 23 August 2011 | Gift into a trust | £334,000 |

He died on 7 June 2016

The lifetime tax was as follows:

(i)

		£
PET 13.5.11:		
Gift		130,000
– AE 11/12		(3,000)
– AE 10/11		(3,000)
PET		124,000

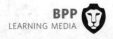

No lifetime tax due on PETs

(ii)

		£
CLT 23.8.11		
Gift		334,000
– AEs (all used)		Nil
CLT		334,000
Less nil band at gift	325,000	
Less GCT's in 7 years before gift	(–)	(325,000)
		9,000
Tax @ 25% ($^{20}/_{80}$)		£2,250

Gross chargeable transfer is £336,250 (334,000 + 2,250)

State the death tax payable on each of the gifts and who it is paid by:

(i) **Gift to daughter**

The tax is £ [   ]

The tax is paid by [▼]

Picklist:

daughter
Mr Raymond's estate
nobody

(ii) **Gift to trust**

The tax is £ [   ]

The tax is paid by [▼]

Picklist:

Mr Raymond's estate
nobody
trustees

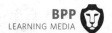

Activity 6: Death tax on lifetime gifts 3

Marco made the following gifts during his lifetime:

15 September 2008	Gross chargeable transfer	£186,000
23 August 2011	Gift to daughter	£164,000

He died on 23 November 2016.

The tax paid by his daughter is £ [   ]

4 Death tax paid on assets owned at death (death estate)

The final stage is to calculate tax payable on the assets owned at death, the death estate.

Step 1

Identify the value of the death estate.

Step 2

Apply exemptions – remember that assets transferred to a spouse/civil partner and gifts to charities and political parties are always exempt. The other exemptions we considered will not apply on death, they are for lifetime transfers only.

Step 3

Identify **all** transfers (PETs and CLTs) made in the seven years prior to death. Deduct the gross value of these transfers from the nil rate band.

Step 4

If there is any nil rate band remaining deduct it from the value of the death estate. Apply the death rate at 40%. The tax is paid out of the value in the estate so the final party named in the will **(the residuary legatee)** effectively pays the tax as they will receive a smaller legacy as a result of the tax payment. The tax is actually paid over by the **executors**, the people responsible for distributing the assets in accordance with the terms of the will.

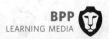

4.1 Calculating the death estate

Illustration 10: The death estate proforma

X Deceased

Date of death .....

	£	£
Freehold property	X	
Less mortgage and accrued interest	(X)	
		X
Stocks and shares		X
Insurance policy proceeds		X
Leasehold property		X
Cars		X
Personal chattels		X
Debts due to deceased		X
Cash		X
		X
Less: debts due from deceased		(X)
funeral expenses		(X)
Less exempt transfers		(X)
CHARGEABLE ESTATE		X

Note: Debts may only be deducted if they are legally enforceable so for example a simple (gratuitous) promise to pay a friend or relative would not be deductible.

Reasonable funeral expenses would also include the cost of a grave stone.

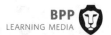

Illustration 11: The death estate

Zack died on 19 June 2016.

Zack's assets at the date of his death consisted of the following.

- 10,000 shares in A plc valued at £8,525
- Cash in bank £9,280
- Freehold property valued at £150,000 subject to a repayment mortgage of £45,000

Zack's debts due at the date of his death were as follows:

- Electricity £150
- Council tax £300

Zack had also told his daughter on 10 June 2016 that he would pay £1,000 towards the cost of her summer holiday and that he would pay her this amount on 1 July 2016.

Zack's executors paid reasonable funeral expenses of £2,000 (including the cost of a tombstone) on 1 September 2016.

Zack's death estate for IHT purposes is as follows:

	£	£
A plc shares		8,525
Cash in bank		9,280
Freehold property	150,000	
Less repayment mortgage	(45,000)	
		105,000
Gross estate		122,805
Less debts and funeral expenses		
electricity (incurred for consideration)	150	
council tax (imposed by law)	300	
amount towards holiday for daughter (gratuitous promise)	0	
funeral expenses	2,000	
		(2,450)
Death estate		120,355

4.2 Calculating the tax

Illustration 12: Calculating the death tax on the estate

Zack (above) died on 19 June 2016 and had a taxable estate on death of £120,355. He made the following lifetime gifts:

15 January 2008 CLT – gross chargeable transfer £100,000

27 April 2010 – gift to wife of £30,000

20 June 2014 CLT – £50,000

25 December 2015 PET – £200,000

The inheritance tax on his estate is as follows:

	£	£
Death estate		120,355
Nil band	325,000	
Less gifts made in the previous seven years		
20 June 2014	(50,000)	
25 December 2015	(200,000)	
Taxable at 0%		(75,000)
Taxable at 40%		45,355
IHT payable		18,142

Activity 7: Tax on the death estate

Rory died on 5 May 2016, leaving an estate comprising:

- 10,000 ABC plc shares, valued at £24,400
- House worth £350,000
- Summer cottage valued at £84,000
- 1,000 XYZ Investment Ltd shares valued at £68,000

Rory had an outstanding loan of £5,750 at the time of his death.

Rory left a will directing that his son should take the shares, the house should go to his wife and the rest of his estate should go to his daughter. He had made one gross chargeable transfer during his lifetime in 2010 of £232,000.

Rory's chargeable estate is £ _____

The tax on Rory's estate is £ _____

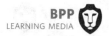

4.3 Spouses/civil partners – transfer of unused nil rate band

If a spouse or civil partner has already died, but didn't use all of their nil band on death, the percentage of nil band unused can be transferred across to the other spouse (or civil partner).

This is not automatic, a claim has to be made.

Illustration 13: Transfer of unused nil rate band

Robert and Claudia were married for many years until the death of Robert on 10 April 2016. In his will, Robert left his death estate valued at £100,000 to his sister. He had made no lifetime transfers.

Claudia died on 12 January 2017 leaving a death estate worth £850,000 to her brother. Claudia had made a chargeable lifetime transfer of £50,000 in 2012.

The inheritance tax payable on the death of Claudia, assuming that a claim is made to transfer Robert's unused nil rate band, is calculated as follows:

	£	£
Claudia's nil rate band	325,000	
Less lifetime transfers	(50,000)	
Remaining nil band		275,000
Robert's nil band	325,000	
Nil band used by Robert at death	(100,000)	
Remaining nil band		225,000
Total nil band available on Claudia's death		500,000

The tax on Claudia's estate is therefore as follows:

	IHT £
£500,000 × 0%	0
£350,000 × 40%	140,000
£850,000	140,000

Activity 8: Transfer of nil rate band

George died on 1 June 2010 with an estate valued at £400,000.

He left £250,000 of his estate to his wife Mildred and the balance to his son.

The nil rate band available for Mildred on her death assuming current rates continue to apply will be £ ⬚

5 Tax planning

Consider the following tax planning points:

- Give assets away during lifetime. This has several benefits:

  – Lifetime exemptions (annual exemption, small gifts etc) can be used

  – If the donor survives seven years there will be no death tax

  – If the donor does not survive seven years but survives at least three then taper relief will be available

- Avoid giving assets to trust if possible as this will result in an immediate charge to inheritance tax.

- Use the nil rate band – effectively you get a new nil rate band every seven years so if you do make gifts into a trust keep them below the £325,000 threshold and if you exceed this wait seven years before making further gifts.

- The younger spouse/civil partner should make gifts as they are more likely to survive seven years. Assets could be transferred from the older spouse/civil partner to the younger without any adverse effects as this would be an exempt transfer. The younger could then transfer to the intended recipient.

- Consider skipping a generation – if you gift assets directly to your grandchildren rather than to your children then HMRC cannot tax your children on their death. If you gift to your children and they then gift to your grandchildren (their children) on their death then effectively your wealth is being taxed twice.

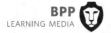

- Inheritance tax is a tax on transfers of wealth.

- The value taxed is the loss to the donor.

- There are three stages to the inheritance tax computation that must be performed in order – lifetime tax on lifetime gifts, death tax on lifetime gifts made in the seven years prior to death and death tax on the death estate.

- There are a number of exemptions available on lifetime gifts the most important being the annual exemption.

- Transfers between spouses/civil partners are always exempt.

- A lifetime transfer is a potentially exempt transfer (PET) if it is a gift to a person or a chargeable lifetime transfer (CLT) if it is a gift to a trust.

- CLTs are taxable during lifetime. PETs are not taxable during lifetime.

- The first £325,000 of taxable gifts are taxable at 0% but this nil band is reduced by any taxable gifts made in the previous seven years.

- CLTs are taxed at rate of 20% if the donee pays the tax but at 20/80 if the donor pays. If the donor pays then the gift must be grossed up by the tax paid.

- All gifts made in the seven years prior to death are chargeable to death tax at 40% including PETs. PETs made in the seven years prior to death will reduce the nil band for future gifts but PETs made more than seven years prior to death can be ignored.

- Gifts made less than seven years before death but more than three years can be tapered. Lifetime tax can be deducted from the death tax.

- Assets held at death (the death estate) are taxed at 40%. The nil rate band can be applied here but it is reduced by chargeable gifts made in the seven years prior to death.

- If someone dies without using their full nil band any unused balance can be transferred to their spouse/civil partner on their death.

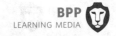

Keywords

- **Annual exemption**: the amount a taxpayer can give away in a tax year without incurring an inheritance tax charge. This is £3,000. Unused annual exemption may be carried forward into the following tax year and used after the current year's.

- **Chargeable lifetime transfer:** a gift to a trust. Tax is immediately payable and also payable again if the donor dies within seven years of making the gift.

- **Nil rate band:** the first £325,000 of chargeable gifts are taxed at a rate of 0%. Gifts made in the previous seven years will reduce the nil rate band.

- **Potentially exempt transfer**: a gift to an individual. There is no tax payable here unless the donor dies within seven years of making the gift.

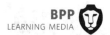

Activity 1: Diminution of value

What is the value of the gift for inheritance tax purposes? £ | 170,000 |

Workings:

IHT:	£
Value before transfer	370,000
Value after transfer	(200,000)
Transfer of value for IHT	170,000

Activity 2: Calculating life time tax – CLTs only

(a) The trust agrees to pay the tax

The tax payable is £ | 23,200 |

The gross chargeable transfer is £ | 331,000 |

Workings:

		£
Gift (CLT)		337,000
AE: 2016/17		(3,000)
2015/16 b/f		(3,000)
Net gift after exemptions		331,000
Nil band left	325,000	
Less GCTs in previous 7 years before gift	(110,000)	(215,000)
		116,000
Tax at 20%		23,200

Gross chargeable transfer is £331,000.

(b) Mr Butcher pays the tax.

The tax payable is £ | 29,000 |

The gross chargeable transfer is £ | 360,000 |

Workings:

	£	£
Net gift after exemptions, as before		331,000
– Nil band left	325,000	
Less: GCTs in 7 years before gift	(110,000)	
		(215,000)
		116,000
Tax at 25% (20/80)		29,000

Gross chargeable transfer is £360,000 (331,000 + 29,000).

Activity 3: Calculating lifetime tax – PETs and CLTs

(i)   Gift to daughter

The tax is £ | nil |

(ii) Gift to trust

The tax is £ | 3,000 |

(iii) Gift to son

The tax is £ | nil |

Workings:

	£
Gift to daughter 15.3.16	
Gift	50,000
AE: 2015/16	(3,000)
2014/15 b/f	(3,000)
PET	44,000
No lifetime tax	

	£
Gift to trust 13.8.16:	
Gift	343,000
AE: 2016/17	(3,000)
2015/16 already used	–
Gross CLT	340,000
Less nil band left	(325,000)
	15,000
Tax @ 20%	3,000
GCT £340,000	
Gift to son 19.8.16	
Gift	30,000
AE: 2016/17 and 2015/16 already used	–
PET	30,000

No lifetime tax.

Activity 4: Death tax on lifetime gifts 1

(i) Gift to nephew

The tax is £ | nil |

The tax is paid by | nobody |

(ii) Gift to granddaughter

The tax is £ | nil |

The tax is paid by | nobody |

(iii) Gift to son

The tax is £ | 12,600 |

The tax is paid by | son |

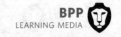

Workings

Lifetime tax:

None as all transfers are PETs

Death tax:

	£	£
(i) PET March 2009		
– more than 7 years before death ∴ exempt		
(ii) PET October 2013:		
Gift		158,000
– Marriage exemption		(2,500)
– AE 13/14		(3,000)
– AE 12/13 b/f		(3,000)
PET		£149,500
< nil band (£325,000) ∴ no tax due		
GCT		£149,500
(iii) PET November 2014:		
Gift		210,000
– AE 2014/15		(3,000)
PET		207,000
Less nil band left	325,000	
Less GCT's in 7 years before gift	(149,500)	
		(175,500)
		31,500
Tax @ 40%		£12,600
Payable by the son		
(No taper relief as <3 years before death)		

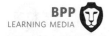

Activity 5: Death tax on lifetime gifts 2

(i) Gift to daughter

The tax is £ | nil |

The tax is paid by | nobody |

(ii) Gift to trust

The tax is £ | 30,210 |

The tax is paid by | trustees |

Workings:

Death tax:

		£	£
(i)	PET 13.5.11		124,000
	< nil band at death (£325,000) ∴ no death tax		
	GCT		£124,000
(ii)	CLT 23.8.11		336,250
	Less nil band left	325,000	
	Less GCT's in 7 years before gift	(124,000)	
			(201,000)
			135,250
	Tax @ 40%		54,100
	Less taper relief (4–5 years) 40%		(21,640)
	Less lifetime tax		(2,250)
	Additional tax on death		£30,210
	Payable by Trustees		

Activity 6: Death tax on lifetime gifts 3

The tax paid by his daughter is £ | 3,040 |

Workings:

	£	£
15.9.2008 – no further tax as donor survived 7 years		
23.8.2011 Gift – PET becomes chargeable		158,000
(164,000 – 6,000)		
Less:		
Nil band remaining	325,000	
Less GCTs in 7 years before **gift**	(186,000)	
		(139,000)
		19,000
Tax @ 40%		£7,600
Less taper relief: 5–6 years: 60%		(4,560)
IHT due		£3,040

Activity 7: Tax on the death estate

Rory's chargeable estate is £ | 170,650 |

The tax on Rory's estate is £ | 31,060 |

Workings:

Death Estate

	£	£
ABC plc shares		24,400
House	350,000	
– exempt as left to spouse	(350,000)	
Summer cottage		84,000
XYZ Ltd shares		68,000
		176,400

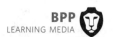

	£	£
Less liabilities		(5,750)
Chargeable estate		170,650
Less nil band remaining		
Nil band at date of death	325,000	
– used in 7 years before death	(232,000)	
		(93,000)
		77,650
Tax @ 40%		£31,060

Activity 8: Transfer of nil rate band

The nil rate band available for Mildred on Mildred's death assuming current rates continue to apply will be £ 500.000

Workings:

	£
Mildred's own nil band	325,000
Unused nil band of husband	175,000
	500,000
George's estate	400,000
Less exempt transfer	(250,000)
Using up nil band	150,000
Nil rate band unused 325,000 – 150,000 = 175,000	

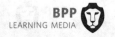

Test your learning

1   Gillian owned a 70% shareholding in R Ltd, an unquoted investment company. On 23 July 2016, she gave a 20% shareholding in R Ltd to her son. The values of shareholdings in R Ltd on 23 July 2016 were as follows:

	£
100% shareholding	600,000
70% shareholding	350,000
50% shareholding	200,000
20% shareholding	80,000

What is the diminution in value of Gillian's estate as a result of her gift on 23 July 2016?

Tick ONE box.

	✓
£150,000	
£270,000	
£80,000	
£120,000	

2   Joel and Sunita were a married couple. Sunita died in July 2009 and 65% of her nil rate band of £325,000 (2009/10) was unused. Joel died in May 2016. He had made a potentially exempt transfer (after all available exemptions) of £75,000 in August 2012. Joel left his estate to his sister. Any relevant elections were made.

What is the nil rate band available to set against Joel's death estate?

Tick ONE box.

	✓
£325,000	
£452,800	
£461,250	
£536,250	

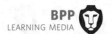

3   On 7 July 2011, Paul made a gross chargeable transfer (after all exemptions) of £260,000. On 19 December 2016 he gave £190,000 to a trust. Paul agreed to pay any lifetime IHT due.

How much inheritance tax will be payable by Paul on the December 2016 transfer of value?

Tick ONE box.

	✓
£28,250	
£31,250	
£29,750	
£23,800	

4   Donald made the following transactions in the tax year 2016/17:

(1)   A gift of £2,000 to his grand-daughter on the occasion of her marriage.

(2)   A sale of a vase to his friend, Alan, for £1,000 which both Donald and Alan believed to be the market value of the vase. The vase was later valued by an auction house as worth £20,000 at the date of the sale.

Ignoring the annual exemption, what is the total value of potentially exempt transfers made by Donald as a result of these gifts?

Tick ONE box.

	✓
£21,000	
Nil	
£2,000	
£19,000	

5   Kirstin gave shares worth £150,000 to a trust on 15 September 2009 and shares
     worth £600,000 to her brother on 10 July 2013. Kirstin died on 23 October 2016.
     These figures are stated after claiming the relevant annual exemptions.

     What is the inheritance tax payable on Kirstin's death in relation to her lifetime
     transfers?

Tick ONE box.

	✓
£170,000	
£88,000	
£136,000	
£132,160	

6   Mary made the following gifts in the tax year 2016/17:

     (1)   £1,000 on the first day of each month for nine months to her grand-son to pay
           university living expenses. Mary used income surplus to her living requirements
           to make these payments.

     (2)   £100 to her grand-nephew on his birthday and a further £250 to the same
           grand-nephew as a Christmas gift.

     Ignoring the annual exemption, what is the total value of potentially exempt transfers
     made by Mary as a result of these gifts?

Tick ONE box.

	✓
£9,350	
£100	
£9,000	
£350	

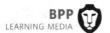

7 Daniel owned all 1,000 shares in Q Ltd, an unquoted investment company. On 10 October 2016, Daniel gave 300 of his shares in Q Ltd to his daughter. The values of the shares on 10 October 2016 were as follows:

% shareholding	Value per share £
76 – 100	150
51 – 75	120
26 – 50	90
1 – 25	30

What is the diminution in value of Daniel's estate as a result of his gift on 10 October 2016?

Tick ONE box.

	✓
£123,000	
£27,000	
£66,000	
£18,000	

8 Susanna died on 19 November 2016. Her estate consisted of a house worth £200,000 (on which there was a repayment mortgage of £60,000) and investments and cash totalling £350,000. Her executors paid funeral expenses of £5,000. Susanna left a cash legacy of £100,000 to her husband and the residue of her estate to her son and daughter. Susanna had not made any lifetime transfers of value.

How much inheritance tax will be payable on Susanna's estate?

£ [ ]

9 Rodney died on 13 August 2016. In his will he left £200 in cash to each of his five nephews, investments held in ISAs valued at £350,000 to his daughter, and the residue of his estate, which amounted to £520,000, to his wife.

What is the chargeable estate for inheritance purposes?

£ [ ]

10 Ruth made a chargeable lifetime transfer of £750,000 on 18 June 2016. The tax rate used was 20/80. Ruth died on 10 July 2016.

Who pays the lifetime tax and the death tax?

Tick ONE box.

Lifetime tax	Death tax	✓
Ruth	Ruth's estate	
Ruth	Trustees	
Trustees	Ruths's estate	
Trustees	Trustees	

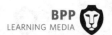

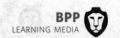

Employment income

4

Learning outcomes

2	Calculate a UK taxpayer's total income
2.1	Calculate income from employment
	• Calculate employment income, including salaries, wages, commissions and bonuses
	• Calculate taxable benefits in kind
	• Identify exempt benefits in kind
	• Identify and calculate allowable and exempt expenses
3	Calculate income tax and National Insurance (NI) contributions payable by a UK taxpayer
3.2	Apply relief for pension payments and charitable donations
	• Apply occupational pension schemes
	• Apply private pension schemes
	• Apply charitable donations
3.5	Advise on tax planning techniques to minimise tax liabilities
	• Maximise relevant exemptions and reliefs
	• Change benefits in kind to make them more tax efficient
	• Change investment incomes to make them more tax efficient
	• Make other changes that can minimise tax liabilities

Assessment context

Benefits are highly examinable. Make sure you can calculate and explain them. In the initial AAT sample assessment Task 2 tested the rules on car benefits for 8 marks. Task 3 tested other benefits for 8 marks. Task 6 required you to perform a detailed income tax calculation for 12 marks and so in your assessment a brief employment income working could form part of this task. Task 8 tested a number of sundry matters for 7 marks, one of the questions related to quantifying the difference in tax an employee would pay if they chose one benefit over another.

Qualification context

You will not see the information in this chapter outside of this unit.

Business context

You will not see these areas again in your AAT qualification outside of this unit.

Chapter overview

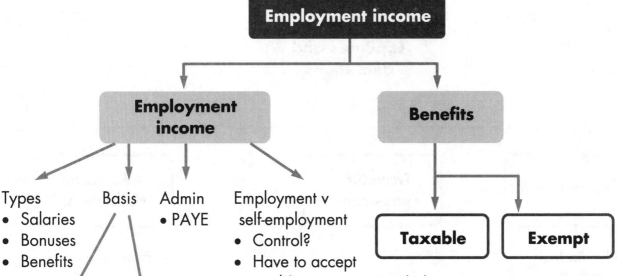

Employment income

Employment income

Benefits

Types
- Salaries
- Bonuses
- Benefits

Basis

Admin
- PAYE

Employment v self-employment
- Control?
- Have to accept work?
- Provide further work?
- Provide equipment?
- Hire helpers?
- Risk?
- Responsibility?
- Opportunity to profit?
- Work when choose?
- Wording?

Taxable

See below

Exempt

- Job-related accommodation
- Canteen
- Removal exp (£8,000)
- Car parking
- Pool cars
- Nurseries
- £55/£28/£25 per week childcare
- Employer pension contributions
- Sports facilities
- Counselling on redundancy
- Staff parties (max £150)
- Incidental expenses (£5/£10)
- Mileage allowance
- Mobile phones
- £4/week home working
- Bus subsidies
- Buses
- Bicycles
- Long service awards
- Staff suggestion schemes
- Air miles
- Training
- Taxis
- £500 medical expenses
- £250 third-party gifts
- Gifts outside of employment
- Payment or reimbursement of allowable business expenses

Normal rules
Earlier of
- Earned
- Received

Rules for directors
Earlier of
- Payment
- Entitlement
- Credited in accounts
- AP end if determined before AP end
- Date determined if after AP end

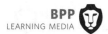

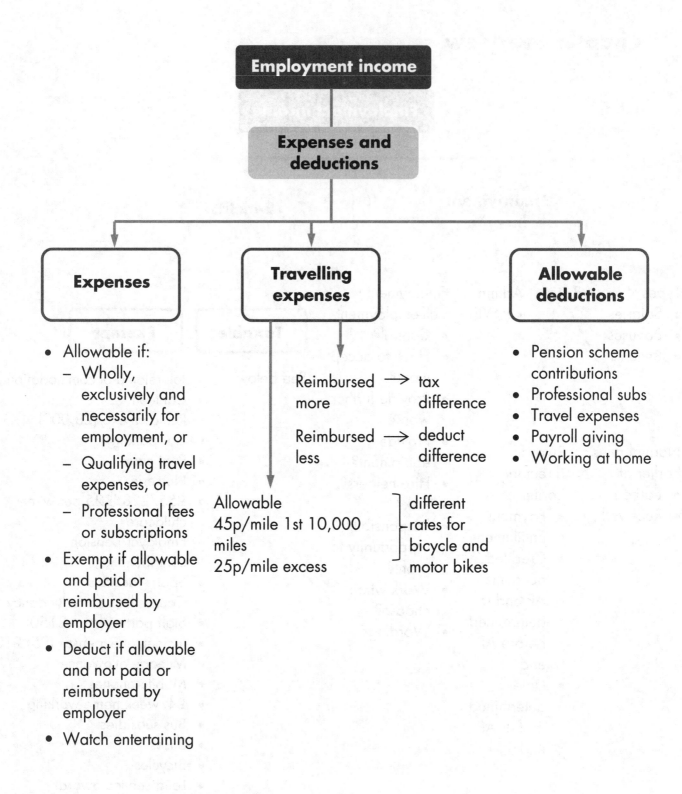

Employment income

Expenses and deductions

Expenses

- Allowable if:
  - Wholly, exclusively and necessarily for employment, or
  - Qualifying travel expenses, or
  - Professional fees or subscriptions
- Exempt if allowable and paid or reimbursed by employer
- Deduct if allowable and not paid or reimbursed by employer
- Watch entertaining

Travelling expenses

Reimbursed more → tax difference

Reimbursed less → deduct difference

Allowable
45p/mile 1st 10,000 miles
25p/mile excess

different rates for bicycle and motor bikes

Allowable deductions

- Pension scheme contributions
- Professional subs
- Travel expenses
- Payroll giving
- Working at home

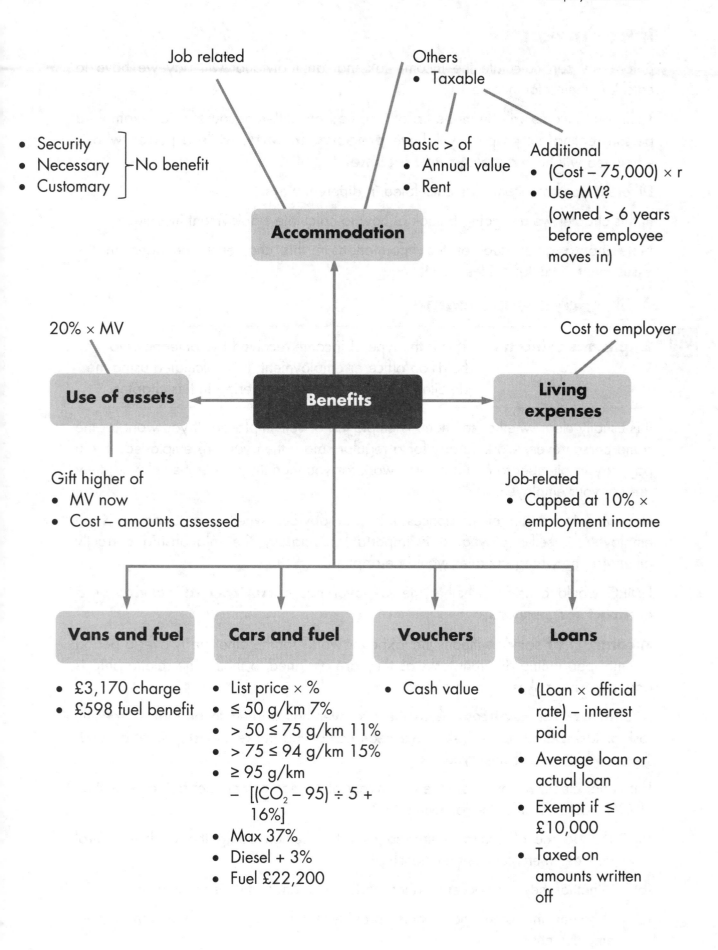

Job related

Others
- Taxable

- Security
- Necessary ⎤ No benefit
- Customary ⎦

Basic > of
- Annual value
- Rent

Additional
- (Cost − 75,000) × r
- Use MV?
  (owned > 6 years
  before employee
  moves in)

Accommodation

20% × MV

Cost to employer

Use of assets ← **Benefits** → **Living expenses**

Gift higher of
- MV now
- Cost − amounts assessed

Job-related
- Capped at 10% ×
  employment income

Vans and fuel

- £3,170 charge
- £598 fuel benefit

Cars and fuel

- List price × %
- ≤ 50 g/km 7%
- > 50 ≤ 75 g/km 11%
- > 75 ≤ 94 g/km 15%
- ≥ 95 g/km
  − [(CO_2 − 95) ÷ 5 +
    16%]
- Max 37%
- Diesel + 3%
- Fuel £22,200

Vouchers

- Cash value

Loans

- (Loan × official
  rate) − interest
  paid
- Average loan or
  actual loan
- Exempt if ≤
  £10,000
- Taxed on
  amounts written

Introduction

Before we can calculate the income tax that an individual will pay we have to calculate their total income.

Their total income will be made up of income from different sources; for example a person renting out property will have **property income**, while a person who is employed will have **employment income**.

Different types of income are calculated in different ways.

In this chapter we are going to look at how to calculate employment income.

Note that a great deal of the information in this chapter is provided in the assessment in the tax tables.

1 Employment income

> **Employment income** This is the type of income received by someone who holds an office or employment. It is calculated using the detailed rules we will be considering in this chapter.

It is usually clear whether someone is employed or self-employed. If you work for the same person every working day for a regular salary then you are employed. If you pay, say, a plumber to perform some work for you then they are self-employed; they are not your employee.

However, in certain circumstances it is not obvious whether a taxpayer is an employee or self-employed. It is important to classify the relationship correctly otherwise the wrong tax rules would be applied.

HMRC would consider whether the taxpayer has a **contract of service** or **a contract for services**.

A contract of service means the taxpayer works for the other party over a period of time, performing different tasks as they are assigned to them. The relationship is ongoing. This makes them employed.

A contract for services means the taxpayer has agreed to perform a specific task or tasks. Once these tasks have been completed the relationship is at an end. This makes them self-employed.

If it is not clear whether we have a contract of service or contract for services then HMRC would consider the following:

(a) The degree of control exercised over the person doing the work – control implies an employment relationship

(b) Whether they must accept further work – obligation implies employment

(c) Whether the other party must provide further work – obligation implies employment

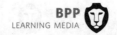

(d) Whether they provide their own equipment – using someone else's equipment implies an employment relationship

(e) Whether they hire their own helpers – hiring their own helpers suggests autonomy meaning they are self-employed

(f) What degree of financial risk they take – self-employment is more risky than employment

(g) What degree of responsibility for investment and management they have – self-employed people have more responsibility than employed people

(h) Whether they can profit from sound management – self-employed people will benefit directly from good decisions they make

(i) Whether they can work when they choose – self-employed people have more flexibility over how they work

(j) The wording used in any agreement between the parties – this will help us to understand the nature of the relationship

In this unit we are only concerned with the taxation of employed people. The calculation of income from self-employment is a major part of the *Business Tax* syllabus.

2 Taxation of employment income

2.1 Types of income

A taxpayer will be taxed on any amounts deriving from an office or employment performed wholly or partly in the UK including:

- Salaries, bonuses and commissions
- Non-cash benefits, for example a company car
- Payments made on termination of employment

2.2 Basis of assessment

These rules identify the tax year that income is taxed in. There are normal rules and additional rules that apply to directors only.

2.2.1 Normal rules

A taxpayer will be assessed on amounts received in the current tax year (6 April 2016 – 5 April 2017).

Earnings are treated as received at the earlier of:

- The time when payment is made
- The time when a person becomes entitled to payment of the earnings

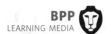

Illustration 1: Basis of assessment

Joy is employed by R plc. She is entitled to the payment of a bonus of £2,000 on 31 March 2017, although she does not receive it until 25 April 2017.

Joy will be taxed on the bonus in 2016/17 because she is entitled to payment on 31 March 2017.

Activity 1: Basis of assessment

Rudolph is an employee of Mabuse Ltd. He earns a salary of £28,000 but on 1 November 2016 he is promoted and his salary increases to £35,000. The company also pays him a bonus relating to the year ended 31 March 2016 of £3,000 on 15 May 2016. The bonus for the year ended 31 March 2017 of £4,000 is paid on 13 May 2017.

Required

(a) What is Rudolph's taxable salary for 2016/17?

£ ☐

(b) What is Rudolph's taxable bonus for 2016/17?

£ ☐

2.2.2 Rules for directors

Special rules apply to company directors. Their earnings are treated as being received on the earliest of:

- The time when payment is made
- The time when a person becomes entitled to payment of the earnings
- The time when the amount is credited in the company's accounting records
- The end of the company's period of account (if the amount has been determined by then)
- The time the amount is determined (if after the end of the company's period of account)

2.3 Deduction of tax by employers

Employers have an obligation to deduct income tax from payments they make to their employees under the **Pay As You Earn (PAYE) system**. Tax is deducted on both cash payments and benefits. Employees therefore receive their salary net of tax.

Most employees will have the correct amount of tax deducted by their employers so there will be no need for them to complete a tax return or make further payments of tax.

In your assessment salaries will be quoted gross. This means you are given the figure before tax has been deducted. You will then be provided with information as to the amount of income tax deducted under PAYE.

3 Taxable benefits

Certain perks provided by employers represent **benefits** taxable on employees. The rules on these are set out in legislation called the **benefits code**.

There are specific rules applying to certain benefits, for example cars. If there is no specific rule then employees will be taxed on the cost to the employer of providing the benefit.

As a general rule:

- There is no taxable benefit if there is no private benefit to the employee (eg no benefit for the use of a projector in class by a BPP tutor)

- Time apportion the benefit if it is not available for the whole tax year

- Deduct any contributions made by the employee from the benefit

3.1 Cars

A car provided by the employer that is available for private use gives rise to a benefit. If fuel is provided for private motoring there will be an additional benefit.

Note that HMRC considers commuting to work and back as private use so in practice if an employee uses a car belonging to their employer they will normally be taxed on this as a benefit. The exception to this would be a **pool car** (see later).

3.1.1 Car benefit

The starting point for calculating a car benefit is the list price of the car. A percentage of that list price is the taxable benefit.

The price of the car is calculated as follows:

- List price when new, plus optional extras costing at least £100
- Deduct capital contributions made by employee (capped at £5,000)

The percentage used varies, depending on the CO_2 emissions and whether the car is petrol- or diesel-fuelled.

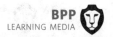

Assessment focus point

CO$_2$ g/km	Petrol engine	Diesel engine
≤ 50 g/km	7%	10%
> 50 ≤ 75 g/km	11%	14%
> 75 ≤ 94 g/km	15%	18%
≥ 95 g/km	Calculation • Minimum 16% • Maximum 37%	Calculation • Minimum 19% • Maximum 37%

The rate for electric cars is always 7%.

Formula provided

For cars that emit CO$_2$ of more than 94 g/km, the taxable benefit percentage starts at 16% and increases by 1% for every 5 g/km (rounded down to the nearest multiple of 5) by which CO$_2$ emissions exceed 95 g/km, up to a maximum of 37%.

Illustration 2: Car benefit percentage

Working for a car with CO$_2$ emissions > 94 g/km

The relevant CO$_2$ percentage for a petrol car with 187 g/km CO$_2$ emissions is calculated as follows:

Round down to 185

185 – 95 = 90

Divided by 5 = 18

Add basic 18 + 16 = 34%

Diesel cars have a supplement of 3%. The maximum benefit, however, remains 37% of the list price.

The benefit is apportioned if the car is not available for the whole year or cannot be used for a period of at least 30 days (for example if being repaired).

The benefit is reduced by any payment the user must make for the private use of the car (as distinct from a one-off capital contribution to the cost of the car which would be deducted from the price before applying the percentage).

Pool cars are exempt. A car is a pool car if all the following conditions are satisfied:

- It is used by more than one employee/director and not ordinarily used by one of them to the exclusion of others.

- Any private use is incidental to business use.

- Not normally kept overnight at or near the residence of an employee.

3.1.2 Fuel benefit

Where fuel is provided for private miles (including commuting) there is a further benefit in addition to the car benefit.

The taxable benefit is a percentage of a base figure. The base figure for 2016/17 is £22,200 (see tax tables).

The percentage is the same percentage as is used to calculate the car benefit.

Assessment focus point

Exceptionally there is no reduction in benefit for contributions made by the employee – don't get caught out by this!

There is no benefit if the employee pays for all private fuel.

Illustration 3: Car and fuel benefit

An employee was provided with a new petrol engine car costing £15,000 (the list price) on 6 June 2016. During 2016/17, the employer spent £900 on insurance, repairs and the vehicle licence. The firm paid for all petrol (£2,300) without reimbursement. The employee was required to pay the firm £25 per month for the private use of the car. The car has CO_2 emissions of 84 g/km.

The total taxable benefit for 2016/17 in respect of the car and fuel is calculated as follows:

	£
List price £15,000 × 15%	2,250
£2,250 × 10/12	1,875
Less contribution (10 × £25)	(250)
	1,625
Fuel benefit £22,200 × 15% × 10/12	2,775
Total taxable benefit	4,400

If the contribution of £25 per month had been towards the petrol, the contribution would not be deducted, making the benefit assessable £250 greater. Conversely, if the cost of private petrol was fully reimbursed by the employee, then there would have been no fuel benefit at all.

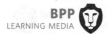

Activity 2: Car and fuel benefit

Damon who works for Stuart Ltd earns £50,000 (PAYE £21,000) and has use of a company car, a Jaguar S-Type 2.5 (brand new). The CO_2 emissions rate is 169 g/km. The car has a list price of £60,000 but the employer negotiated a discount and bought it for £57,000. The company fitted accessories (CD player and child safety seat) at a cost of £900.

Damon is required to pay £100 per month towards the running costs of the car (excluding petrol). The company meets all Damon's petrol costs in 2016/17 which amounted to £3,500.

Required

(a)   What is Damon's taxable benefit for 2016/17?

£ _____

(b)   What is the benefit if Damon left the company on 1 January 2017 and returned the car on that date? £ _____

3.2 Vans

There is a £3,170 charge when vans are available to employees for private use.

Assessment focus point

Note that, unlike company cars, a home to work journey does not qualify as private use for a van.

If the van has CO_2 emissions of 0, then the benefit is 20% of the normal benefit ie £634.

There is an additional £598 charge if fuel is made available for private use.

3.3 Other assets

The following rules apply if any other asset is provided to an employee.

3.3.1 Use of asset

Formula to learn

If an employee is allowed to use an asset owned by their employer for private purposes they will be assessed on the higher of:

- 20% of the value when first made available to employee
- Rental paid by employer

3.3.2 Gift of asset

Formula to learn

If an employee is given an asset that previously belonged to their employer they will be assessed as follows:

- If already used by employee, the higher of:
  - Market value when given
  - Original value when first used less values already assessed

- If a new asset is given, then the employee will be assessed on the cost of providing the asset

- If the asset is a computer, the benefit can only be current market value

- Deduct from the benefit any payment the employee makes for the asset

Illustration 4: Use and gift of asset

A suit costing £200 is bought by an employer for use by an employee on 6 April 2015. On 6 April 2016, the suit is purchased by the employee for £15, its market value then being £25.

The benefit taxable in 2015/16 will be 20% × £200 = £40

The benefit taxable in 2016/17 will be the greater of:

(a) Market value at acquisition by employee = £25

(b)

	£	£
Original market value	200	
Less assessed in respect of use 2015/16	(40)	
	160	
Therefore (b)		160
Less price paid by employee		(15)
Taxable benefit 2016/17		145

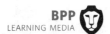

Activity 3: Use and gift of employer's asset

Gustav Holst, an employee, was given the use of some video equipment on 6 October 2014, when it had a value of £1,000. On 6 January 2017, he was given the asset outright when it was worth £500.

Required

Complete the following:

In 2016/17, his benefit for the use of the asset is £ _____

In 2016/17, his benefit on the gift of the asset is £ _____

3.4 Beneficial loans

There is a benefit when an employer gives an employee an interest-free loan or when the employer charges less than a commercial interest rate.

The benefit is the difference between the interest that should have been charged, using the official rate of interest (given in the exam), and the interest paid by the employee.

Formula to learn

Where the size of the loan has changed during the year, the interest is calculated on either of the following:

- The average loan outstanding in the year
- The loan outstanding on a month by month basis

The average method is usually used but either the taxpayer or HMRC can elect to use the month by month calculation.

There is no benefit if the total of all loans made to the employee in the year is £10,000 or less. If this limit is broken then all loans are taxed, not just the excess over £10,000.

An employee will always be taxed on the value of a loan written off by the employer even if the loan was below the £10,000 limit.

Illustration 5: Beneficial loan

At 6 April 2016, a low interest loan of £30,000 was outstanding to a director, who repaid £20,000 on 6 January 2017. The remaining balance of £10,000 was outstanding at 5 April 2017. Interest paid during the year was £250.

The benefit under both methods for 2016/17, assuming that the official rate of interest was 3% throughout 2016/17, is calculated as follows:

Average method

	£
$3\% \times \dfrac{(30,000 + 10,000)}{2}$	600
Less interest paid	(250)
Taxable benefit	350

Alternative method

	£
£30,000 × 9/12 × 3%	675
(6 April 2016 – 6 January 2017)	
£10,000 × 3/12 × 3%	75
(7 January 2017 – 5 April 2017)	
	750
Less interest paid	(250)
Taxable benefit	500

Therefore, the taxable benefit will be £350.

Activity 4: Beneficial loan

At 6 April 2016, a taxable cheap loan of £30,000 was outstanding to an employee earning £12,000 a year, who repaid £20,000 on 7 December 2016. The remaining balance of £10,000 was outstanding at 5 April 2017. Interest paid during the year was £250.

The official rate of interest was 3%.

Required

Complete the following sentences:

The benefit calculated under the average method is £ ☐

The benefit calculated under the strict method is £ ☐

The taxpayer would be taxed on £ ☐

3.5 Accommodation

3.5.1 Job-related accommodation

An employee who is provided with **job-related accommodation** will not be taxed on it under the benefit rules.

Key term

Job-related accommodation	is that which is: • Provided for security reasons, for example for the Prime Minister; or • Necessary for the proper performance of duties, for example a caretaker; or • Customary for that sort of work and ensures better performance of duties, for example a pub landlord would traditionally be provided with accommodation.

3.5.2 Accommodation that is not job related

If the accommodation is not job-related, then a taxable benefit arises on employees and is calculated in two stages:

(1)   The basic charge is calculated as:

Formula to learn

Basic charge – greater of:

• Annual value
• Rent paid by employer

Illustration 6: Accommodation rented by employer

Tony is provided with a company flat:

	£
Annual value	3,000
Rent paid by the company	3,380
Amount paid by Tony to the company for the use of the flat	520

Tony's taxable benefit is:

	£
Benefit: greater of:	
(a) Annual value	3,000
(b) Rent paid by the company	3,380
Therefore	3,380
Less reimbursed to the company	(520)
Net benefit	2,860

(2)   There is an additional charge if the employer owns the building and the cost of the property is greater than £75,000. This is calculated as:

Formula to learn

Accommodation additional charge: (Cost – 75,000) × official rate of interest

Illustration 7: Accommodation owned by employer

Simon's employer provided him with a house throughout 2016/17. The company bought the house for £133,000 on 1 April 2012.

For 2016/17, the annual value of the house is £1,400. Simon pays £3,000 for the use of the house to his employer.

The total benefit arising in respect of the house for 2016/17, assuming the official rate of interest is 3%, is:

Basic charge:

	£
Annual value	1,400
Less Simon's contribution	(1,400)
	Nil

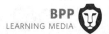

Additional charge:

	£	£
Cost	133,000	
Less	(75,000)	
Excess		58,000
£58,000 × 3%		1,740
Less Simon's contribution (£3,000 – 1,400)		(1,600)
Total benefit 2016/17		140

(3) If the accommodation was acquired more than six years before it was provided to an employee, then the additional charge is based on the market value at the start of the tax year in which the employee moves in.

Activity 5: Accommodation benefit

Ralph has the use of a house belonging to his employer, for which he pays a nominal rent of £2,500. The annual value is £3,000. Ralph has lived in the house since October 2000. It had cost the company £175,000 in October 1999 but is now worth £300,000.

Take the official rate of interest at 3%.

Required

(a) **What is the benefit if the accommodation is job related?**

£ ⬚

(b) **What is the benefit if the accommodation is not job related?**

£ ⬚

(c) **What is the benefit if the accommodation is not job related but was bought in October 1992?**

£ ⬚

3.5.3 Accommodation living expenses

A benefit arises on an employee if their household living expenses are paid for by their employer.

The benefit depends on the accommodation provided:

Formula to learn

- Job-related accommodation:

  Lower of

  – Cost of expenses to employer
  – 10% × net earnings (ie employment income including all other benefits)

- Not job related:

  – Cost of expenses to employer

Expenses include the following items:

- Heating, lighting, cleaning etc
- Repairing, maintaining or decorating
- Providing furniture (annual value taken as 20% of cost)

Activity 6: Accommodation living expenses

Maggie lives in accommodation provided by her employer and her salary is £7,000 per year. Household expenses of £1,800 are paid by her employer and she has other benefits totalling £2,000.

Required

Complete the following sentences:

If the property is 'job related' her benefit is £ ⬚

If the property is not 'job related' her benefit is £ ⬚

3.6 Vouchers

The employee is normally taxed on the cost incurred by the employer in providing a voucher or credit token (for example a credit card).

If the employee receives a cash voucher, a voucher that can be exchanged for cash, they are taxed on the amount that the voucher can be exchanged for.

Certain vouchers are exempt (see below).

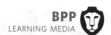

4 Exempt benefits

The following benefits are not taxable. Much of this information is provided in the reference material and tax tables in the assessment.

(a)   Job-related accommodation.

(b)   Canteen offering free or discounted food available to all staff. A benefit would arise if the canteen was only available to selected staff members. The benefit would be the cost to the company net of payments made by the employee.

(c)   Qualifying removal expenses up to £8,000 when the employee has to move house because of their job. Qualifying costs include legal and removal costs as well as purchasing replacement goods such as curtains and carpets. Excess payments over the £8,000 would be taxable.

(d)   Car parking spaces near place of work.

(e)   Occasional taxi fares home where employees are required to work late after 9:00pm.

(f)   Use of pool cars.

(g)   Workplace nurseries (crèches). The crèche must be operated by the employer.

(h)   If the employer pays for the worker's childcare provided by an external provider then some of the payment will be tax free but any excess over a weekly threshold will be taxable. The employer could pay the childcare provider directly or give the employee vouchers. The limits are £55 per week for a basic rate taxpayer, £28 for a higher rate taxpayer and £25 per week for an additional rate taxpayer.

(i)   Contributions by an employer into an approved pension scheme.

(j)   Sport and recreational facilities available generally for the staff. These must be provided directly by the employer. If the employer pays for facilities provided by an external supplier then this will create a taxable benefit.

(k)   Outplacement counselling services to employees made redundant who have been employed full-time for at least two years. The services can include counselling to help adjust to the loss of the job and to help in finding other work.

(l)   Annual staff events up to a maximum of £150 per head. If this limit is exceeded then the full cost is taxable.

(m)   Incidental expense of £5 per night if working away from home (telephone calls, laundry etc). The limit is £10 if working abroad. These amounts may be aggregated if working away a number of days; for example, if working away for 3 days then the limit for the period would be £15.

(n)   Mileage allowances (see later).

(o)   Mobile phones – these are exempt if a single phone is provided. A benefit would apply to additional phones provided to the employee.

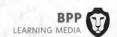

(p) £4 per week may be paid tax free to cover the cost of home working when the employee is required to work from home. Greater amounts may be claimed if the taxpayer can produce evidence of the actual costs incurred by working from home.

(q) Subsidies paid to bus services used by employees for commuting.

(r) Provision of buses for nine or more employees for commuting.

(s) Provision of bicycles and cycling safety equipment for commuting.

(t) Non-cash gifts given to employees as a reward for service in excess of 20 years are exempt provided the cost is no more than £50 per year worked.

(u) Awards under staff suggestion schemes.

(v) Air miles obtained by business travel.

(w) Work-related training.

(x) Medical treatment of up to £500 to assist an employee to return to work.

(y) 'Goodwill' gifts of up to £250 from a single third party.

(z) Gifts made to employees outside of employment, for example a marriage gift.

5 Allowable deductions

Certain expenses may be deducted from employment income before tax is applied.

Assessment focus point

The general rule for allowable deductions states that expenses must be incurred **'wholly, exclusively and necessarily'** (HMRC, 2014) in the performance of duties. This means that if the employee could perform their duties without incurring the expense then it is not deductible as it is not strictly necessary.

The following are specific allowable deductions:

- Fees and subscriptions to relevant professional bodies

- Travelling and other expenses incurred in the performance of duties

- Contributions to an approved occupational pension scheme; an occupational scheme is one provided by the employer

- Donations to charity under **payroll deduction scheme**

- £4 per week deduction to cover household expenses incurred when working at home

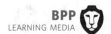

5.1 Expenses

Employees will incur expenditure performing their job. They may or may not be reimbursed by their employer for these expenses. Certain business expenses are allowable:

- Wholly, exclusively and necessarily incurred in the performance of the duties of the employment, or

- Qualifying travel expenses (see 5.1.4), or

- Professional fees and subscriptions

The treatment of these expenses depends upon whether the employee is reimbursed for the expenditure by their employer or not.

5.1.1 Employee incurs expenditure without reimbursement

If the employee bears the cost of the expense themselves without reimbursement from their employer then they would simply deduct the expense from their employment income.

Illustration 8: Expenses not reimbursed

Paul earns a salary of £35,000 a year. He has to pay his £500 subscription to the Chartered Institute of Taxation. Paul's employer does not reimburse him for this expense.

Paul's employment income calculation would be as follows:

	£
Salary	35,000
Less expenses	(500)
Employment income	34,500

5.1.2 Employee incurs expenditure and is reimbursed by employer, or employer pays directly

From 2016/17 the payment or reimbursement of expenses is exempt (ie no need to include in earnings) if they are fully allowable and the employee would therefore otherwise be able to claim a deduction. Employers will no longer be required to apply for a dispensation. This makes the administration of such expenses far simpler.

Illustration 9: Reimbursed expenses

Paul earns a salary of £35,000 a year. His employer reimburses him for his £500 subscription to the Chartered Institute of Taxation.

The subscription is exempt income as it is a reimbursed allowable expense, so it is not included in the calculations of earnings.

	£
Salary	35,000
Reimbursed expenses (exempt)	nil
Employment income	35,000

5.1.3 Expenses with a private and business element

Strictly, if an expense has a 'private' and 'business' component, then it is not exclusively used in the duties of employment and will not be allowed (for example if a phone is used for work purposes and privately, then no deduction can be claimed for the line rental, although the cost of the business calls would be allowed).

In practice, HMRC will allow taxpayers to apportion costs where there is a business and a private element. The business use will be an allowable expense, and deductible for the employee on their tax return. If the allowable element is clearly identifiable, the exemption will apply.

5.1.4 Travel expenses

Travelling expenses are deductible; if the employer reimburses this is an exempt benefit. As noted above, if expenses are not reimbursed then the taxpayer may deduct the expense.

Only business travelling is allowable. Normal commuting from home to office is not included.

An exception is where an employee is seconded to a **temporary workplace** for less than 24 months; here commuting from home is allowable.

5.1.5 Approved mileage allowance payments

Employers may reimburse employees for using their own car on their employer's business. The reimbursement is to cover fuel and all other costs associated with using the car, for example depreciation, road tax and insurance.

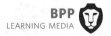

Formula provided

The allowable limits are:

- 45p per mile for the first 10,000 miles per tax year
- 25p per mile for the excess

If the employer pays more than the permitted amount, the excess is taxable.

If the employer pays less than the permitted amount, the employee can deduct the difference from their earnings.

There are separate rates for motorcycles and bicycles. These would be given to you in the exam.

Illustration 10: Statutory mileage

Owen drives 14,000 business miles in 2016/17 using his own car.

You are required to calculate the taxable benefit/allowable deduction assuming:

(a) He is reimbursed 45p a mile
(b) He is reimbursed 25p a mile

	£
Statutory limit: 10,000 × 45p	4,500
4,000 × 25p	1,000
	5,500

(a)

	£
Amount received (14,000 × 45p)	6,300
Less statutory limit	(5,500)
Taxable benefit	800

(b)

	£
Amount received (14,000 × 25p)	3,500
Less statutory limit	(5,500)
Allowable deduction	(2,000)

Activity 7: Statutory mileage

Jen drives 15,000 miles in the tax year.

Required

(a) Choose the correct option and insert the numerical value.

If Jen's employer pays her 30p per mile she

may deduct	is taxed on	£

(b) Choose the correct option and insert the numerical value.

If Jen's employer pays her 50p per mile, she

may deduct	is taxed on	£

5.1.6 Entertaining customers

If an employee spends money entertaining customers or clients and claims reimbursement, the normal rules seen above will apply.

Rather than reimbursing specific expenses, an employer may simply give an employee an annual allowance to cover expenses. As this is effectively additional salary, it is taxable but the employee may claim a deduction for expenses actually incurred.

The exception to this is an employee may not claim a deduction against a round sum allowance for entertaining costs.

This is because the employer is claiming a deduction against their profits for paying the employee the allowance. Normally, a business cannot claim a deduction for entertaining costs. If the employee is allowed to escape taxation on this part of the allowance, then effectively customers are being entertained with no tax consequences for the employer or employee.

5.2 Contributing to a pension

An employee may save tax by paying into a pension.

5.2.1 Maximum contributions

Formula to learn

The maximum tax relief available for pension contributions each year is the higher of:

- £3,600
- Earnings for the year

Additional contributions are permitted but no tax relief will be available on these.

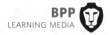

5.2.2 Tax relief

Effectively the taxpayer's income is being reduced by the payment into the pension scheme so they are no longer paying tax on the top level of their income. They therefore save the tax they would have paid on this income. This saving may be at 20%, 40% or 45% depending on their level of income. A 20% taxpayer saves tax of 20p for every £1.00 contribution, a 40% taxpayer saves tax at 40p for every £1.00, while a 45% taxpayer would save 45p for every £1.00.

The method of relief is different depending on the type of pension scheme.

Key term

Personal pension scheme	A personal pension scheme is organised by the taxpayer. Contributions are made net of basic rate tax (20%). Additional relief is available for higher and additional rate taxpayers by **extending the basic rate band**. This is identical to the way taxpayers get relief for Gift Aid payments and we will consider this in detail in Chapter 7 – Calculation of income tax.
Occupational scheme	An occupational scheme is one provided by an employer. Contributions are deducted directly from earnings. PAYE is then applied to just the remaining income. This is called a **net pay arrangement**.

5.2.3 Employer contributions

An employer may also contribute to either an occupational scheme or a personal scheme on behalf of the employee.

Employer contributions are not taxable benefits on the employee.

There is no limit on the amount of contributions an employer can make.

5.3 Donations to charity

Employees may request that their employer pays some of their salary to an approved charity of their choice.

The donation is deducted from gross salary before PAYE is applied. It therefore saves the taxpayer tax at their highest marginal rate of tax.

This is sometimes called '**Give-As-You-Earn**' or **GAYE**.

6 Tax planning

There are a number of ways an employee can legally reduce their income from employment:

- Select exempt benefits over taxable benefits

- Select benefits with a lower cash equivalent over benefits with a higher cash equivalent

- Ensure that any contribution towards the private use of an employer's car is for the use itself as this would be deductible rather than for the private fuel which would not be deductible

- Pay into a company pension scheme

- Make payments to charity under the payroll giving scheme

- Claim all allowable deductions, for example the £4 a week allowance for home working

- Avoid overtime working if this will take their income over £100,000 leading to a reduction in the personal allowance and a significant increase in tax (see later)

- Seek rewards in benefits rather than in cash as there will be no National Insurance cost to the employee on benefits (note the employer would have to pay National Insurance here).

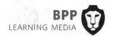

Chapter summary

- It is important to distinguish between income from employment and self-employment. The basic question is whether the person is employed under a contract of service, or performs services under a contract for services.

- An employee's earnings comprise wages or salary and bonuses and benefits.

- Money earnings are received on the earlier of the time payment is made and when the employee becomes entitled to payment. There are special rules for directors.

- The taxable benefit on a car is a percentage of the car's list price. This varies with carbon dioxide emissions. There is an additional benefit if fuel is provided.

- The private use of a pool car is an exempt benefit.

- There is a taxable benefit for private use of a van (but home to work travel is not treated as private use) plus a further benefit if private fuel is provided.

- If the employer provides the employee with assets for private use, there is a taxable benefit each year of 20% of the value of the assets when first provided.

- Employer loans written off give rise to a taxable benefit. For loans there is a benefit equal to the excess of official rate of interest over interest actually charged.

- The living accommodation benefit is based on the annual value of the property. An additional benefit arises where the cost of the property exceeds £75,000.

- Expenses incurred by the employer in connection with the provision of living accommodation are fully assessable on the employee, unless the employee is in job-related accommodation in which case the benefit is restricted.

- There are certain exempt benefits which are not taxable on employees.

- A deduction is given to employees for using their own vehicle for business travel if any mileage allowance paid is less than the statutory rates. Any excess is taxable.

- Employees are generally allowed a deduction for travel costs incurred in the performance of their duties, or incurred in travelling to and from home to a temporary workplace. Temporary is taken to be not exceeding 24 months.

- Occupational pension schemes are employer-run schemes. No taxable benefit arises in respect of employer contributions made to pension schemes.

- Employee contributions to an occupational pension scheme are deducted from the employee's taxable earnings before tax is applied.

- Individuals can make pension contributions up to the higher of:

  - The basic limit (£3,600 – 2015/16)
  - Earnings

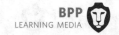

- Employees can make charitable donations under an employer's payroll deduction scheme. Such payments are deductible in arriving at taxable earnings.

- For other employment-related expenses to be deductible, such expenses must be 'wholly, exclusively and necessarily' (HMRC, 2014) incurred 'in the performance of' the employee's duties.

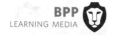

Keywords

- **Approved mileage allowance payments scheme:** lays down authorised mileage rates (AMR) at which employees may claim an allowance for business journeys made in their own car

- **Job-related accommodation:** accommodation that is either necessary for the proper performance of duties, or for the better performance of the employee's duties and is customarily provided in that type of employment, or is provided as part of special security arrangements

- **Net pay arrangements:** where an employer deducts an employee's occupational pension contributions from the employee's earnings before they deduct income tax

- **Payroll deduction scheme:** set up by an employer to enable employees to make tax-deductible donations to charity

- **Temporary workplace:** one at which the employee expects to be for no more than 24 months

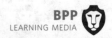

Activity answers

Activity 1: Basis of assessment

(a)

£ | 30,916

(b)

£ | 3,000

Workings

	£
Salary:	
6 April 2016 to 31 October 2016 – $\frac{7}{12}$ x 28,000	16,333
1 November 2016 to 5 April 2017 – $\frac{5}{12}$ x 35,000	14,583
Total salary	30,916
Bonus received between 6 April 2016 and 5 April 2017	3,000

Activity 2: Car and fuel benefit

(a)

£ | 23,730

Workings

	£
List price + accessories (60,000 + 900)	60,900
30%(W) x £60,900	18,270
Less employee contributions (12 x £100)	(1,200)
Car benefit	17,070
Plus fuel benefit (£22,200 x 30%)	6,660
Total benefit	23,730

(W)	Round down to 165	
	Relevant emissions percentage:	
	165 – 95 =	70
	Divide by 5 =	14
	Add basic	16
		30%

(b)

£ | 17,798

Workings (not provided in the CBT)

	£
$30\% \times £60{,}900 \times \dfrac{9}{12}$	13,703
Less employee contributions (9 × £100)	(900)
Car benefit	12,803
Add fuel benefit ($£22{,}200 \times 30\% \times \dfrac{9}{12}$)	4,995
Total benefit	17,798
Alternatively – $23{,}730 \times \dfrac{9}{12}$	17,798

Activity 3: Use and gift of employer's asset

In 2016/17, his benefit for the use of the asset is £ | 150

In 2016/17, his benefit on the gift of the asset is £ | 550

Workings

Use of employer's assets

	£	£
2014/15 Use: $20\% \times 1,000 \times \dfrac{6}{12}$	100	
2015/16 Use: $20\% \times 1,000$	200	
2016/17 Use: $20\% \times 1,000 \times \dfrac{9}{12}$	150	
		450

Gift

	£	£
2016/17 Higher of:		
• Value when given	500	
• Value when first made available for use less already		
Assessed (1,000 – 450)	550	
le		550

Activity 4: Beneficial loan

The benefit calculated under the average method is £ | 350 |

The benefit calculated under the strict method is £ | 450 |

The taxpayer would be taxed on £ | 350 |

Workings

Average method	£
$3\% \times \dfrac{30,000 + 10,000}{2}$	600
Less interest paid	(250)
Benefit	350

Alternative method (strict method)	£
£30,000 × $\frac{8}{12}$ (6 April – 6 December) × 3%	600
£10,000 × $\frac{4}{12}$ (7 December – 5 April) × 3%	100
	700
Less interest paid	(250)
Benefit	450

The taxpayer would not opt for the strict method.

HMRC may opt for the alternative method if it suspects tax avoidance.

Activity 5: Accommodation benefit

(a) £ [nil]

(b) £ [3,500]

(c) £ [7,250]

Workings

Accommodation (house bought in 1999)	£
Annual value	3,000
Less rent paid	(2,500)
	500
Add 3% × (175,000 – 75,000)	3,000
Taxable benefit	3,500

The property was less than six years old when Ralph moved in so the benefit is based on cost.

Accommodation (house bought in 1992)	£
Annual value	3,000
Less rent paid	(2,500)
	500
Add 3% × (300,000 – 75,000)	6,750
Taxable benefit	7,250

The property was more than six years old when Ralph moved in so the benefit is based on market value.

Activity 6: Accommodation living expenses

If the property is 'job related' her benefit is £ | 900 |

If the property is not 'job related' her benefit is £ | 1,800 |

Workings

Living expenses	£
Lower of:	
(a) Living expenses	1,800
(b) 10% of net earnings:	
= 10% (7,000 + 2,000)	900
Taxable benefit	= 900

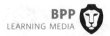

Activity 7: Statutory mileage

(a) If Jen's employer pays her 30p per mile she

may deduct	£1,250

Working

Mileage calculation			£
Receives	15,000 × 0.30		4,500
Approved HMRC rates	10,000 × 0.45	4,500	
	5,000 × 0.25	1,250	(5,750)
Deductible			(1,250)

(b) If Jen's employer pays her 50p per mile she

is taxed on	£1,750

Working

Mileage calculation		£
Receives	15,000 × 0.50	7,500
Approved HMRC rates	(as above)	(5,750)
Taxable		1,750

Test your learning

1   **Fill in the missing words.**

Someone is regarded as self-employed if they have a contract [   ] ,
whereas if they have a contract [   ], they will be regarded as an employee.

2   **Fill in the missing words.**

Expenses are allowable if they are incurred [   ], [   ] and
[   ] in the performance of the duties of employment.

3   Brian uses his own car to travel 8,000 business miles in 2016/17. Brian's employer
reimburses him with 35p per mile travelled. The approved mileage rate for the first
10,000 business miles travelled is 45p per mile.

**The amounts that are taxable(deductible) in calculating employment
income are (both minus signs and brackets can be used to indicate
negative numbers):**

£ [   ]

4   An employee is provided with a flat by his employer (not job-related
accommodation). The annual value of the flat is £4,000; rent paid by the employer
amounts to £5,900 per annum.

The taxable value of this benefit for 2016/17 is:

£ [   ]

5   A taxable fuel benefit is reduced by any reimbursement by the employee of the cost
of fuel provided for private mileage.

Tick ONE box.

	✓
True	
False	

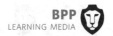

6   A video recorder costing £500 was made available to Gordon by his employer on 6 April 2015. On 6 April 2016, Gordon bought the recorder for £150, when its market value was £325.

The assessable benefit that arises in 2016/17 is:

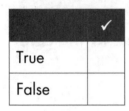

	✓
£325	
£400	
£175	
£250	

7   There is no benefit on the first £10,000 of an interest-free loan.

Tick ONE box.

	✓
True	
False	

8   Gautown was supplied with a petrol engine car by his employer throughout 2016/17. The list price of the car was £24,000 and its CO_2 emissions were 153 g/km.

The taxable benefit arising in respect of the car is:

£ [   ]

9   Buster is the Managing Director of Buster Braces Ltd and is supplied with a Bentley (3 litre, petrol engine) which cost £72,000. It has CO_2 emissions of 165 g/km. All running costs are borne by the company. Buster is also provided with a mobile phone for private and business use. The cost of provision of the phone to Buster Braces Ltd is £750 in 2016/17.

The total taxable benefits are:

£ [   ]

10 **For each of the following benefits, tick whether they would be taxable or exempt if received by an employee in 2016/17:**

Item	Taxable	Exempt
Write off loan of £8,000 (only loan provided)	☐	☐
Payments by employer of £500 per month into registered pension scheme	☐	☐
Provision of one mobile phone	☐	☐
Provision of a company car for both business and private use	☐	☐
Removal costs of £5,000 paid to an employee relocating to another branch	☐	☐
Accommodation provided to enable the employee to spend longer time in the office	☐	☐

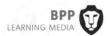

Property income

5

Learning outcomes

2	Calculate a UK taxpayer's total income
2.3	Calculate income from property • Calculate profit and losses from residential furnished and unfurnished property
3	Calculate income tax and National Insurance (NI) contributions payable by a UK taxpayer
3.5	Advise on tax planning techniques to minimise tax liabilities • Maximise relevant exemptions and reliefs • Change investment incomes to make them more tax efficient • Make other changes that can minimise tax liabilities

Assessment context

Task 5 in the initial AAT sample assessment tested the detailed rules on property income for 6 marks. Task 6 required you to produce a detailed income tax calculation and this included a brief working for property income. Task 8 consisted of a number of requirements for 8 marks one of which tested tax planning for a couple with investment income.

Qualification context

You will not see these areas again in your AAT qualification outside of this unit.

Business context

Property may be an additional source of income for some people. For others, it will be their livelihood. Anyone investing in property needs to understand the tax implications.

Chapter overview

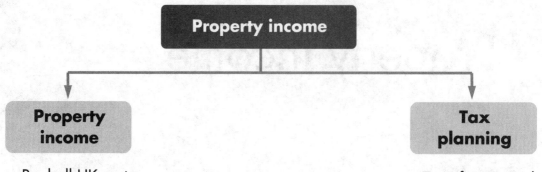

Property income

Property income

- Pool all UK rents
- Rent accruing in tax year
- Deduct expenses (accruals basis)
- Claim relief for replacement of furniture
- Relief for losses

Tax planning

- Transfer ownership of property to spouse paying lower rate of tax

Introduction

Before we can calculate income tax payable for the tax year we need to calculate a taxpayer's total income. This consists of the grand total of their income from various sources. One source of income included in this total would be the income realised from letting out property. This chapter looks at how we calculate this income.

1 Property income

1.1 What is property income?

Property income is all income derived from renting out land and/or buildings.

Key term

Landlord	The person letting out the property.
Tenant	The person letting the property.
Furnished letting	A property furnished by the landlord.
Unfurnished letting	A property in which furniture is provided by the tenant.

Note. The tax rules are different for furnished and unfurnished.

1.2 Basis of assessment

A landlord is assessed on rent accruing in the current tax year from UK properties. This is taxed as non-savings income.

Illustration 1: Accruing rent

Susi bought a property on 6 September 2016. She began letting the property immediately for an annual rent of £36,000 payable in advance in 3-monthly instalments due on 6 September, 6 December, 6 March and 6 June.

Rental income is taxed on an accruals basis. This means the income which arises from the letting for the period between 6 September 2016 and 5 April 2017 is taxed in 2016/17. Susi is therefore taxed on £36,000 × 7/12 = £21,000. She actually receives instalments of £9,000 on 6 September, 6 December and 6 March in the tax year, giving total receipts of £27,000, but this is not relevant for the tax calculation.

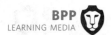

Activity 1: Accruing rent

Len owns a flat in Lancing. He lets it out unfurnished at an annual rental of £6,000 from 1 January 2016. Rent is payable quarterly in advance. On 1 January 2017, he raised the rent to £6,600 per annum.

Required

Calculate the property income for tax year 2016/17.

£ [   ]

1.3 Allowable deductions from property income

The landlord may deduct all incidental expenses, also calculated on an **accruals basis**. These must be revenue in nature, this means regular ongoing costs giving a short-term benefit, for example insurance. Capital costs are not deductible; these are one-off expenses that give a long-term benefit, for example installing central heating.

The following costs would be allowable if paid by the landlord:

- Advertising, accountancy and insurance
- Business rates and council tax
- Bad debts
- Management and agent's fees

If the landlord borrowed money to purchase the property, the interest paid on the loan is deductible as an expense against property income. Note though the actual repayments of the loan cannot be deducted.

1.4 Repair expenditure

Sometimes it is difficult to distinguish between revenue and capital expenses. A good example would be repair costs. If the costs constitute regular costs required to maintain the property in its current condition then these would be allowable, for example decorating and routine maintenance.

If the repair represents an improvement then it is not allowable, for example if the landlord installed a second bathroom in the property. Note also that if the building is bought in a dilapidated state then the initial costs incurred to make it usable again would also be capital and not allowed.

1.5 Furniture

There is no relief available when the landlord first buys furniture and equipment for the property.

When these assets are replaced the landlord may claim the full cost of the replacement in the tax year in which the replacements were bought.

The following assets would qualify for replacement furniture relief:

- Movable furniture or furnishings, such as beds or suites
- Televisions
- Fridges and freezers
- Carpets and floor coverings
- Curtains
- Linen
- Crockery or cutlery
- Beds and other furniture

If an asset is replaced with a better asset then only the cost of a similar replacement would be allowable.

Note that replacement of integral features such as bathrooms and central heating systems would be covered by the repair rules above.

1.6 Capital allowances

Capital allowances may be claimed on plant and machinery used in the letting business (you would be given a figure for this).

Illustration 2: Allowable expenses

Nadine has let a furnished property for many years. The accrued rent for 2016/17 is £41,000.

Expenses relating to the letting were:

	£
Insurance (year to 31 December 2016)	600
Insurance (year to 31 December 2017)	800

In June 2016, the tenant accidentally flooded the bathroom. Nadine took the opportunity to strip out the aged bathroom suite and convert the bathroom into a wet room at a total cost of £5,000. This included £900 that was the cost of repairing the flood damage.

During the year the washing machine broke and Nadine bought a replacement washer/drier for £400. An equivalent washing machine would have cost £300.

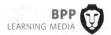

Nadine's property income for 2016/17 is:

	£	£
Rental income		41,000
Less insurance (£600 × 9/12) + (£800 × 3/12)	650	
Replacement furniture relief at cost	300	
Repairs	900	
		(1,850)
Taxable property income		39,150

Note. The rental income and expenses must be dealt with on an accruals basis.

The cost of the flood repairs is allowable because it is a revenue expense. However, the cost of converting the bathroom into a wet room is not allowable because this is a capital expense.

1.7 More than one property – pooling income and expenses

Income and expenses from different properties are pooled to give a single total for property income.

	£
Total property income	X
Total allowable deductions	(X)
Profit/(loss)	X/(X)

Profits and losses on different properties are thus automatically offset.

Illustration 3: Property pooling calculation

Bahrat lets two properties in 2016/17.

Property 1 was bought in June 2016 and let unfurnished from 1 July 2016 at an annual rent of £18,000 per annum. Buildings insurance of £8,000 was paid for the year to 30 June 2017. £1,200 was spent in June 2016 on advertising for tenants.

Property 2 became vacant on 5 April 2016. Bahrat then spent £7,000 on repairing the leaking roof in the property. The unfurnished property was let again with effect from 1 March 2017 for £24,000 per annum, payable monthly in advance. Buildings insurance of £1,800 was incurred for the year to 31 March 2017.

Bahrat's property income for 2016/17 is:

	£	£
Rental income – Property 1 (9/12 × £18,000)		13,500
Rental income – Property 2 (1/12 × £24,000)		2,000
Less: Buildings insurance		
– Property 1 (9/12 × £8,000)	6,000	
– Property 2	1,800	
Advertising for tenants	1,200	
Repairs	7,000	
		(16,000)
Overall property loss		(500)

Pooling income and expenses on all let properties effectively allows a loss on one property to be set against income from other properties.

1.8 Losses

If the overall result is a profit it is taxable in the current year.

If the overall result is a loss carry it forward to use against property income in the future. The loss can carry forward indefinitely until it is used.

Activity 2: Property income

Fiona owns a property that she lets furnished on a short-term basis. In the year ended 5 April 2017, she accrued rents of £8,400 and incurred the following expenses:

	£
Agent's commission	360
Mortgage repayments (including interest of £500)	800
Insurance – year to 31 December 2016	400
– year to 31 December 2017	500
Repairs	1,200

Repairs include £300 to replace a broken window; the balance was to install a brand new window. There had been no window here before but Fiona decided the new window would offer views that would encourage future lettings.

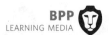

She also replaced a single bed with a double bed. The double bed cost £400. An equivalent single bed would have cost £300.

Fiona has a property loss brought forward of £500.

Required

How much is assessable on her as property income in 2016/17?

£ [   ]

2 Tax planning

Property income is **non-savings** income and is taxed at 20%, 40% or 45% depending on the taxpayer's level of income.

Spouses or civil partners or couples cohabiting or friends or relatives may own property either jointly or individually. One party may be paying tax at a higher rate than the other. If this is the case it makes sense to have the property owned by the taxpayer who is paying tax at the lower rate as they will then receive the income and it will be taxed at a lower rate reducing the overall tax liability.

One party may therefore need to transfer property to another.

Taxpayers with relatively low levels of income have a personal allowance. This represents an amount of income that can be earned before tax is paid. If this personal allowance is not used in the year it is usually lost.

However, if one of the parties has no income then the property should be transferred to them so they can offset their personal allowance against the income. This will enable them to use a personal allowance that would otherwise have been wasted.

Assets including cash can be transferred between spouse and civil partners without causing inheritance tax or capital gains tax problems. If the parties are not married or in a civil partnership it may cause tax issues. For the planning to be effective the asset or cash to buy an asset must be transferred with 'no strings attached', the spouse receiving the asset has total control over it and makes no promises to return the asset at a later date or pay the income generated to the other party. Clearly you must trust the other party before following this course of action!

HMRC will disregard transactions which appear to be artificial and undertaken purely for a tax advantage so for the planning to work there must be some other purpose for the transaction, for example a wife with a husband who is not working could gift a property to him so that he has a source of income of his own and some independence.

Chapter summary

- Property income is all income derived from letting out land and buildings.

- It is calculated on an accruals basis for a tax year and taxed as non-savings income.

- It is net of income and expenditure. Expenditure is allowable if it is for regular ongoing costs, repairs or the replacement of furniture. Capital costs are not allowable.

- Income and expenses on different properties are pooled to give a grand total. A net positive result will be taxable. A net negative result is a loss that may be carried forward and offset against property income in the future.

- Couples should ensure properties are owned by the spouse/civil partner who is paying tax at a lower rate or has an unused personal allowance.

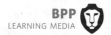

Keywords

- **Accruals basis:** for taxing rental income means that all rent owing or accruing in a tax year is taxed in that year

- **Furnished letting:** a letting which includes the use of furniture belonging to the landlord

- **Landlord:** someone who rents out a property to another person

- **Tenant:** the person who occupies the land or building

- **Unfurnished letting:** a letting just of the property without furniture

Activity answers

Activity 1: Accruing rent

Property income £ [6,150]

Workings (not provided in the CBT)

	£
Rent (6.4.16 – 31.12.16) $6,000 \times \dfrac{9}{12}$ =	4,500
Rent (1.1.17 – 5.4.17) $6,600 \times \dfrac{3}{12}$ =	1,650
Total	6,150

Activity 2: Property income

£ [6,015]

Workings (not provided in the CBT)

	£
Rents	8,400
Less expenses commission	(360)
Replacement cost of equivalent single bed	(300)
Mortgage interest	(500)
Insurance $(\dfrac{9}{12} \times 400) + (\dfrac{3}{12} \times 500)$	(425)
Repairs to existing window	(300)
Property income	6,515
Less property losses brought forward	(500)
	6,015

1   David buys a property for letting on 1 August 2016 and grants a tenancy to Ethel from 1 December 2016 at £3,600 per annum, payable quarterly in advance.

    The rental income taxable in 2016/17 is:

    £ [   ]

2   John pays buildings insurance premiums for 12 months in advance on 1 October each year to cover all his rental properties. He pays £4,800 in 2015 and £5,200 in 2016.

    What amount for building insurance would be allowed against his rental income for 2016/17?

    £ [   ]

3   Harry owns a property which he lets for the first time on 1 July 2016 at a rent of £4,000 per annum, payable monthly in advance.

    The first tenants left on 28 February 2017 and the property was re-let to new tenants on 4 April 2017 at a rent of £5,000 per annum, payable yearly in advance.

    Harry's allowable expenditure was £1,000 in 2016/17.

    What is his taxable rental income for 2016/17?

    £ [   ]

4   Ben and Polly are married. Polly earns a salary of £200,000 a year meaning she pays tax at 45%, Ben has trading income of £20,000 meaning he pays tax at 20%. They are planning to buy an investment property which they will let out for £12,000 a year.

    To minimise their tax liability the property should be [▼]

    Picklist:

    held in Polly's name
    held in Ben's name
    held jointly by Ben and Polly
    held in trust

5   **Property losses may be:**

	✓
Carried back one year and offset against property income only	
Offset against net income in the current year	
Carried forward for one year only and offset against property income	
Carried forward indefinitely and offset against property income only	

Taxable income

6

Learning outcomes

2	Calculate a UK taxpayer's total income
2.2	**Calculate income from investments** • Identify and calculate taxable investment income • Identify exempt investment income
3	**Calculate income tax and National Insurance (NI) contributions payable by a UK taxpayer**
3.1	**Calculate personal allowances** • Calculate personal allowances • Calculate restrictions on personal allowances
3.2	**Apply relief for pension payments and charitable donations** • Apply private pension schemes • Apply charitable donations
3.5	**Advise on tax planning techniques to minimise tax liabilities** • Maximise relevant exemptions and reliefs • Change investment incomes to make them more tax efficient • Make other changes that can minimise tax liabilities

Assessment context

Calculating taxable income is a step on the way to calculating income tax payable which we will consider in Chapter 7. In the initial AAT sample assessment Task 4 tested the rules on investment income seen in this chapter and Chapter 7 for 6 marks. Task 6 required you to perform a detailed income tax calculation using the rules in this chapter and Chapter 7. It also required you to do a separate personal allowance restriction working. 12 marks were available in total. Task 8 consisted of a number of requirements for 8 marks one of which tested tax planning for a couple with investment income, another tested the tax planning technique of paying into a personal pension scheme to reduce net income and thus preserve the personal allowance.

Qualification context

If you are studying *Business Tax* as well as *Personal Tax* then the material in this chapter will be useful background for you in your *Business Tax* studies. However, you will not be tested on the material in this chapter in the *Business Tax* CBT.

Business context

Preparation of taxable income computations forms part of the work a tax adviser will perform for their client.

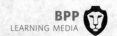

Chapter overview

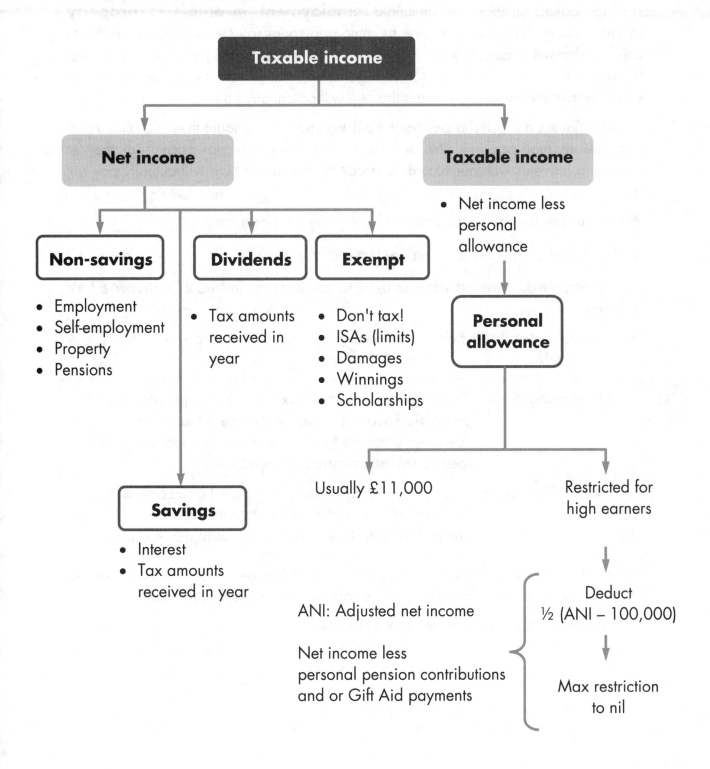

Introduction

Having looked at how to calculate **employment income** and **property income** we are now going to look at some additional sources of income, **savings and dividend income**. We'll also identify some **exempt** income that will never be taxed. We are then going to add together all our sources of income to get our **total or net income**, the amount that we will potentially have to pay tax on.

Most taxpayers are given a **personal allowance**, an amount they are allowed to earn before they pay tax. We will deduct this personal allowance from the net income to leave us with our **taxable income**, the amount we will actually pay tax on.

We'll consider the actual calculation of tax in the following chapter.

1 The income tax computation

The **income tax computation** is used to calculate an individual's **income tax liability**.

The income tax liability is the total amount of income tax the taxpayer is due to pay for the tax year.

Key term

Taxable income	To calculate the income tax liability we apply tax rates to **taxable income**. Taxable income is the grand total of a taxpayer's income from all sources after deducting the **personal allowance**, if applicable.
Personal allowance	The personal allowance is the amount of income a taxpayer is allowed to earn before they pay tax. It can be reduced or withdrawn completely for higher earners.

In this chapter we will calculate taxable income. We will then consider how to calculate the income tax liability on the taxable income in the next chapter.

The calculation of taxable income looks like this:

Assessment focus point

Proforma income tax computation

	Non-savings income £	Savings income (excluding dividends) £	Dividends £	Total £
Employment income	X			X
Property income	X			X
Interest received		X		X
Dividends from UK companies			X	X
Total/net income	X	X	X	X
Less personal allowance	(X)			(X)
Taxable income	X	X	X	X

Note. Total and net income are actually two different concepts but in your syllabus the terms can be used interchangeably. We will use net income for the rest of the chapter.

You will see there are three columns representing three types of income. We will consider the implications of this in the following section.

Some income will be paid over to the taxpayer **net of tax**, meaning tax has already been deducted at source. An example of this would be a salary payment from an employer. This represents an estimate of the tax the taxpayer is likely to have to pay.

We use the income tax computation to calculate the correct amount of tax that a taxpayer should be paying for the year. We therefore need to include all income **gross** of tax, before these estimated amounts of tax have been deducted.

When the tax liability has been calculated then the individual is allowed to deduct the tax already paid for the tax year. This may or may not be the correct amount.

This could leave the taxpayer having to make an additional tax payment or claim a tax repayment.

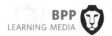

2 Non-savings, savings, dividend and exempt income

Different tax rates apply to the three different types of income:

Key term

Non-savings income	This consists of income from employment, self-employment pensions and property income.
Savings income	This consists of interest received in the tax year.
Dividend income	This consists of dividends received in the tax year.

Note that **exempt income** is income that is never charged to income tax.

2.1 Non-savings income

This is all income other than interest and dividends. It includes the following:

- Income from employment (see Chapter 4 Employment Income)
- Income from property (see Chapter 5 Property Income)
- Income from pensions
- Income from self-employment (the calculation of this income forms part of the *Business Tax* syllabus)

2.2 Savings income

This is interest received. Note it is taxed on an actual basis. If interest is received in the tax year it is taxed. If it is accrued but not received, it is not taxed.

Since 6 April 2016 all interest is received **gross**. There is no longer any requirement for banks and building societies to deduct income tax at source. We simply add together all the interest received in the tax year from all sources and then insert the total into the savings column in the tax computation.

Most taxpayers will not have to pay income tax on interest received unless their interest income is above the **personal savings allowance** (see following chapter).

Illustration 1: Savings income

Gerry receives the following interest:

	£
Lloyds TSB Bank	80
Nationwide Building Society	400
Government interest (gilts)	100

These amounts would be added together to calculate the total interest to be included in the savings column of the tax computation.

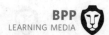

	Gross £
Lloyds TSB Bank	80
Nationwide Building Society	400
Government interest (gilts)	100
Total	580

2.3 Dividend income

From 6 April 2016 dividends are received gross. Before this date the dividend used to be received net.

Taxpayers are taxed on the amount of dividend received in a tax year.

Illustration 2: Dividend income

Maria receives a dividend of £900. This is the gross amount that needs to be included in the computation of net income.

Most taxpayers will not have to pay income tax on dividend received unless their dividend income is above the **dividend allowance** (see following chapter).

2.4 Exempt income

Assessment focus point

Certain income is exempt from income tax. Do not include it in your total of taxable income.

If you are typing in an answer and there is exempt income in the question, state that this is exempt or if there is an exempt box to click, make sure you do this – there will be a mark here.

Exempt income includes the following:

2.4.1 Individual savings accounts (ISAs)

(a)   These are special savings accounts a taxpayer can invest in.

(b)   Individuals may invest up to £15,240 in an individual savings account (ISA) in tax year 2016/17. This could be in the form of cash, shares, unit trusts or insurance policies. Investors may use their entire allowance on one type of investment (eg the whole £15,240 could be invested in cash) or a combination of different investments.

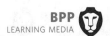

(c) Dividend income from shares and interest income received from cash invested in an ISA are free of income tax. Capital growth is also free of capital gains tax.

(d) An ISA may be opened by someone 16 years old and over if it only contains cash.

(e) ISAs containing investments other than cash may only be opened by someone at least 18 years old.

2.4.2 Others

- Damages awarded as a result of personal injury or death and interest thereon.

- Scholarships/grants, if paid to a student; taxable if paid to their parent as part of their employment income.

- Prizes, lotto winnings, gambling winnings.

- Premium bond prizes.

Activity 1: Taxable and exempt income

Foster receives the following income:

	£
Building society interest	40
Dividend from an ISA investment	900
Rent	6,000
Non-ISA dividends	450

Required

Complete the following table.

Use the picklist options to list the sources of income under the appropriate headings (exempt, non-savings, savings or dividend income).

Record the amounts received under the appropriate column heading (exempt, non-savings, savings and dividends).

You do not need to total the columns.

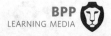

Solution

	Exempt income £	Non-savings income £	Savings income £	Dividend income £
Exempt income				
Non–savings income				
Savings income				
Dividend income				

Picklist:

Building society interest
ISA dividend
Non-ISA dividend
Rent

3 Computation of taxable income

We will now revisit the full income tax computation we looked at in Section 1.

3.1 Net income

In a tax year, all income must be brought together and totalled.

The income is split into three columns representing the three types of income subject to tax:

- Non-savings income
- Savings income
- Dividend income

This gives us net income.

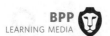

3.2 Taxable income

The personal allowance of £11,000 is then usually deducted from the total/net income to give the taxable amount.

The personal allowance is initially available to all taxpayers, including children.

The personal allowance is reduced for taxpayers who have income in excess of £100,000. The allowance can be potentially reduced to nil.

It is usually most beneficial to deduct the personal allowance against non-savings income before savings income then dividend income.

Illustration 3: Taxable income

In 2016/17, Joe has trade profits of £3,000 and receives bank interest of £17,500 and dividends of £500. Joe's taxable income for 2016/17 is:

	Non-savings income	Savings income	Dividend income	Total
	£	£	£	£
Trade profits	3,000			3,000
Bank interest		17,500		17,500
Dividends			500	500
Net income	3,000	17,500	500	21,000
Less personal allowance	(3,000)	(8,000)	–	(11,000)
Taxable income	–	9,500	500	10,000

Activity 2: Taxable income

Quentin earns a salary of £3,000 in 2016/17. He receives rental income of £1,000, building society interest of £3,750 and a dividend of £5,000.

Required

Prepare a computation of taxable income for 2016/17, clearly showing the distinction between the different types of income.

Solution

	Non-savings income £	Savings income £	Dividend income £	Total £
Employment income				
Property income				
Building society interest				
Dividend income				
Net income				
Less personal allowance				
Taxable income				

4 Restricting the personal allowance

4.1 The basic calculation

If an individual has net income in excess of £100,000 then the personal allowance must be reduced.

It is reduced by £1 for every £2 income the taxpayer has over the £100,000 limit.

The personal allowance may be reduced to £0 if income is greater than or equal to £122,000.

Formula to learn

Restriction = ½ (Net income – 100,000) [limit but no formula given in CBT].

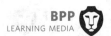

Illustration 4: Personal allowance restriction

In 2016/17, Kelvin has gross employment income of £98,000 and receives building society interest of £1,500 and dividends of £5,000. Kelvin's net income for 2016/17 is:

	Non-savings income £	Savings income £	Dividend income £	Total £
Net income	98,000	1,500	5,000	104,500

The total is above the adjustment threshold of £100,000 so we must reduce the personal allowance.

	£
Net income	104,500
Less income limit	(100,000)
Excess	4,500
Personal allowance	11,000
Less half excess (4,500/2)	(2,250)
Adjusted personal allowance	8,750

The taxable income is therefore:

	Non-savings income £	Savings income £	Dividend income £	Total £
Net income	98,000	1,500	5,000	104,500
Less personal allowance	(8,750)	–	–	(8,750)
Taxable income	89,250	1,500	5,000	95,750

Activity 3: Personal allowance restriction

Karen has net income of £107,000 (all non-savings income).

Required

What personal allowance does Karen receive for 2016/17?

Solution

Her personal allowance is £ [ ]

Her taxable income is £ [ ]

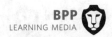

4.2 Charitable donations/pension payments

If a taxpayer makes Gift Aid or personal pension scheme contributions in the year (see next chapter), then they are allowed to deduct the payments from net income before calculating the restriction on the personal allowance.

Both of these payments are made net by the taxpayer but it is the gross amount that is deducted from the net income. We will consider this in detail in the next chapter.

Total income after deducting Gift Aid and personal pension contributions is called **adjusted net income**.

Note. Gift Aid and personal pension contributions are only deducted from total income for the purpose of calculating the personal allowance; they are not deducted from income in the tax computation.

Illustration 5: Personal allowance restriction with Gift Aid payment

As per Illustration 4 in 2016/17, Kelvin has gross employment income of £98,000 and receives building society interest of £1,500 and dividends of £5,000. However, he now makes a gross payment to charity of £1,000 under Gift Aid. Kelvin's net income for 2016/17 is still:

	Non-savings income	Savings income	Dividend income	Total
	£	£	£	£
Net income	98,000	1,500	5,000	104,500

The total is above the adjustment threshold of £100,000 so we must reduce the personal allowance. However, as he has made a payment to charity under Gift Aid we are allowed to reduce the net income before calculating the restriction:

	£
Net income	104,500
Less gross Gift Aid payment	(1,000)
Adjusted net income	103,500
Less income limit	(100,000)
Excess	3,500
Personal allowance	11,000
Less half excess (3,500/2)	(1,750)
Adjusted personal allowance	9,250

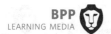

The taxable income is therefore:

	Non-savings income £	Savings income £	Dividend income £	Total £
Net income	98,000	1,500	5,000	104,500
Less personal allowance	(9,250)	–	–	(9,250)
Taxable income	88,750	1,500	5,000	95,250

Activity 4: Personal allowance with personal pension payment

Karen, who has net income of £107,000, now makes a personal pension payment of £2,000 gross.

Required

What personal allowance will Karen receive? What is her taxable income?

Solution

Her personal allowance is £ [   ]

Her taxable income is £ [   ]

We will revisit Gift Aid and personal pension payments in the next chapter.

4 Tax planning

We noted in the previous chapter that married couples/civil partners could minimise their tax liabilities by ensuring that properties being let out were held by the party paying the lower rate of tax or with an unused personal allowance.

The same rule applies here, cash balances yielding interest and shares yielding dividends should be held by taxpayers paying the lower rate of tax or having unused personal allowances.

Other matters to consider:

- Taxpayers could invest in products that yield exempt income such as ISAs or premium bonds.

- Taxpayers could make payments into personal pension schemes or payments to charity under Gift Aid to preserve their entitlement to personal allowance.

Chapter summary

- There are three types of income in the income tax computation: non-savings, savings and dividend.

- Non-savings income includes employment income, property income, trading (or business) income and pension income.

- Savings income is interest received.

- Dividend income is dividends received.

- Exempt income includes income from individual savings accounts (ISAs) and gambling winnings.

- Tax computations must be prepared for a tax year.

- All the components of an individual's income are added together to arrive at 'net income'.

- Net income less the personal allowance gives 'taxable income'.

- The personal allowance is deducted first from non-savings income, then from savings income and finally from dividend income. It is reduced by £1 for every £2 that the individual's net income exceeds the income limit of £100,000.

- The net income figure for comparison to the income limit for the personal allowance is reduced by gross Gift Aid donations and personal pension contributions.

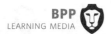

Keywords

- **Dividend income:** dividends received from a company

- **Net income:** an individual's total income calculated prior to deducting the personal allowance

- **Non-savings income:** income other than interest and dividends

- **Personal allowance:** the amount of income a taxpayer may receive before paying tax

- **Savings income:** interest received, for example from a bank or building society

- **Total income:** technically a different sub-total to net income but in your syllabus the terms may be used interchangeably

- **Taxable income:** an individual's net income minus the personal allowance

Activity answers

Activity 1: Taxable and exempt income

	Exempt income £	Non-savings income £	Savings income £	Dividend income £
Exempt income				
ISA dividend	900			
Non–savings income				
Rent		6,000		
Savings income				
Building society interest			40	
Dividend income				
Non-ISA dividend				450

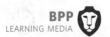

Activity 2: Taxable income

	Non-savings income £	Savings income £	Dividend income £	Total £
Employment income	3,000			3,000
Property income	1,000			1,000
Building society interest		3,750		3,750
Dividend income			5,000	5,000
Net income	4,000	3,750	5,000	12,750
Less personal allowance	(4,000)	(3,750)	(3,250)	(11,000)
Taxable income	nil	nil	1,750	1,750

Activity 3: Personal allowance restriction

Her personal allowance is | £7,500 |

Her taxable income is | £99,500 |

Workings

	£
Personal allowance	11,000
Less ½ (107,000 – 100,000) =	(3,500)
Adjusted personal allowance	7,500
Net income	107,000
Personal allowance	(7,500)
Taxable income	99,500

Activity 4: Personal allowance with personal pension payment

Her personal allowance is | £8,500

Her taxable income is | £98,500

Workings

	£
Net income	107,000
Less personal pension payment	(2,000)
Adjusted net income	105,000
Personal allowance	11,000
Less ½ (105,000 – 100,000)	(2,500)
Adjusted personal allowance	8,500
Net income	107,000
Personal allowance	(8,500)
Taxable income	98,500

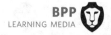

1 **Classify the following types of income by ticking the correct box:**

	Non-savings income	Savings income	Dividend income
Employment income	☐	☐	☐
Dividends	☐	☐	☐
Property income	☐	☐	☐
Bank interest	☐	☐	☐
Pension income	☐	☐	☐
Interest on government stock	☐	☐	☐

2 **Complete the table below to show the amount of income that would be included in a tax return for 2016/17. If your answer is zero, please put a '0'.**

	Amount received £	Amount in tax return £
Building society interest	240	
Interest on an individual savings account	40	
Dividends	160	
Interest from government gilts	350	

3 In 2016/17, Joe has employment income of £30,000 and receives dividends of £300 and premium bond winnings of £500.

Use the table below to show his taxable income for 2016/17.

	Non-savings income £	Dividend income £	Total £

4   Pratish receives property income of £3,000 and building society interest of £9,000 in 2016/17.

Use the table below to show his taxable income for 2016/17.

	Non-savings income £	Savings income £	Total £

5   Jesse has employment income of £112,200 in 2016/17. He also received building society interest of £5,000, a prize of £50 in an internet competition and dividends of £4,000.

Use the table below to show Jesse's taxable income for 2016/17.

	Non-savings income £	Savings income £	Dividend income £	Total £

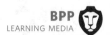

Calculation of income tax

7

Learning outcomes

3	Calculate income tax and National Insurance (NI) contributions payable by a UK taxpayer
3.2	**Apply relief for pension payments and charitable donations** • Apply occupational pension schemes • Apply private pension schemes • Apply charitable donations
3.3	**Perform income tax computations** • Calculate income tax, combining all income into one schedule • Apply tax rates and bands • Deduct income tax at source
3.5	**Advise on tax planning techniques to minimise tax liabilities** • Maximise relevant exemptions and reliefs • Change investment incomes to make them more tax efficient • Make other changes that can minimise tax liabilities

Assessment context

Task 6 of the initial AAT sample assessment required you to perform a detailed income tax calculation as well do a separate question on personal allowance restriction. 12 marks were available.

Qualification context

If you are studying *Business Tax*, then the material in this chapter will be useful background but you will not be tested on these areas outside of this unit.

Business context

Calculating income tax payable is the main task a tax adviser will perform for their client.

Chapter overview

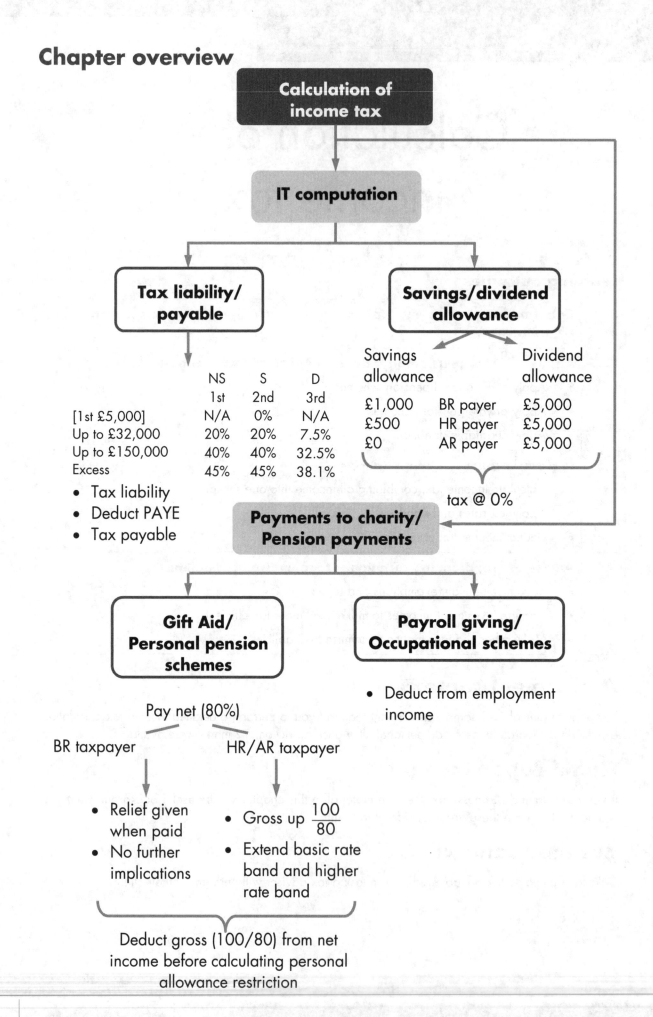

Calculation of income tax

IT computation

Tax liability/ payable

	NS	S	D
	1st	2nd	3rd
[1st £5,000]	N/A	0%	N/A
Up to £32,000	20%	20%	7.5%
Up to £150,000	40%	40%	32.5%
Excess	45%	45%	38.1%

- Tax liability
- Deduct PAYE
- Tax payable

Savings/dividend allowance

Savings allowance   Dividend allowance

£1,000	BR payer	£5,000
£500	HR payer	£5,000
£0	AR payer	£5,000

tax @ 0%

Payments to charity/ Pension payments

Gift Aid/ Personal pension schemes

Payroll giving/ Occupational schemes

- Deduct from employment income

Pay net (80%)

BR taxpayer   HR/AR taxpayer

- Relief given when paid
- No further implications

- Gross up $\frac{100}{80}$
- Extend basic rate band and higher rate band

Deduct gross (100/80) from net income before calculating personal allowance restriction

Introduction

The calculation of income tax will appear complex at first. There is a set of basic rules but these can be applied in many different combinations depending on a taxpayer's circumstances, meaning there are many different scenarios for you to get to grips with.

In this chapter we will consider some but not all of the possible scenarios. The more examples you study and questions you attempt the more familiar you will become with how the rules operate.

1 Calculation of income tax liability

Income tax is calculated at different rates depending on the type and level of income the taxpayer has.

The various rates for 2016/17 are summarised in the diagram below. This data will be provided for you in the taxation tables in your assessment.

The taxable income we calculated in the previous chapter is taxed in the following order:

(1) Non-savings income
(2) Savings income
(3) Dividend income

So, on the diagram we move from left to right.

Illustration 1: Calculation of tax liability

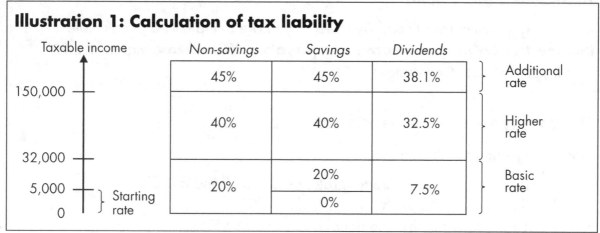

Note we have different **tax bands**.

The **starting rate band** covers taxable income from £1 to £5,000 but only applies to savings income.

The basic rate band covers income from £1 to £32,000. Note the starting rate band forms the first £5,000 of the basic rate band. The starting rate only applies to taxpayers who have less than £5,000 taxable non-savings income so in most calculations it will be ignored.

The **higher rate band** covers income from £32,001 to £150,000.

The **additional rate band** covers income over £150,000.

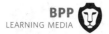

These bands may be adjusted for taxpayers who make payments to charity under Gift Aid or pay into a personal pension scheme.

In addition to these bands, there is a **personal savings allowance** that applies to savings income and a **dividend allowance** that applies to dividend income.

We apply these rates to give us our **income tax liability**.

Income tax liability   The total amount of tax that should be paid on our income.

Key term

Don't forget that an employed taxpayer will have had income tax deducted from their salary before it has been paid to them. This represents an estimated prepayment of income tax for the year. We deduct this from the income tax liability to see whether there is any further **income tax payable** for the year.

It is possible that the taxpayer has paid too much tax. If they have there will be **income tax repayable**.

Income tax payable   Outstanding income tax due for the tax year.

Key term

Income tax repayable   Income tax due to the taxpayer because they have overpaid.

Assessment focus point

Read the requirement very carefully to see if you are being asked to calculate **income tax liability** or **income tax payable**. You will lose marks or waste time if you calculate the wrong one.

2 Taxation of non-savings income

Non-savings income is taxed first.

- It is taxed initially in the starting rate/basic rate band at 20%.
- It is then taxed in the higher rate band at 40%.
- Finally it is taxed in the additional rate band at 45%.

Illustration 2: Non-saving income

Nathan has taxable income of £185,000 consisting entirely of non-savings employment income. PAYE of £65,000 has been deducted.

The non-savings income uses all the basic rate band of £32,000, the next £118,000 of income falls into the higher rate band and the excess above that falls into the additional rate band.

The income tax liability is:

	Income tax £
Non-savings income	
32,000 × 20%	6,400
118,000 × 40%	47,200
150,000	
35,000 × 45%	15,750
185,000	
Income tax liability	69,350
Less PAYE	(65,000)
Income tax payable	4,350

This can be illustrated on the diagram as follows:

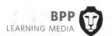

Taxable income	Non-savings	Savings	Dividends	
150,000	45%	45%	38.1%	} Additional rate
	40%	40%	32.5%	} Higher rate
32,000	20%	20%	7.5%	} Basic rate
5,000		0%		
0	} Starting rate			

3 Savings income

Once we have taxed non-savings income we then move on to tax savings income.

We begin taxing savings income in the bands at the point where we finished taxing the non-savings income. So in the previous illustration (Illustration 2) Nathan would pay tax on any savings income in the additional rate band as he has already used his basic rate and higher rate band.

Savings income is taxed as follows:

- At 0% on any savings falling in the starting rate band
- At 20% on any savings falling in the basic rate band
- At 40% on any savings falling in the higher rate band
- At 45% on any savings falling in the additional rate band

However, there is a further complication in that taxpayers will potentially receive the **personal savings allowance**. This represents savings income that is taxed at 0%. Taxpayers receive the personal savings allowance as follows:

A basic rate taxpayer (one who has adjusted net income of less than £43,000) receives a personal savings allowance of £1,000.

A higher rate taxpayer (one who has adjusted net income greater than £43,000 but no more than £150,000) receives a personal savings allowance of £500.

An additional rate taxpayer (one who has adjusted net income greater than £150,000) does not receive a personal savings allowance.

(You will note these thresholds represent the relevant bands plus the personal allowance where this is available so for example the basic rate test equals £32,000 plus £11,000 equals £43,000, the higher rate test equals £150,000 plus £0 as no personal allowance would be available for a taxpayer with £150,000 worth of income.)

Illustration 3: Savings income example 1

Sasha has net income of £41,120 (before the personal allowance) and taxable income of £30,120. Of this, £18,920 is non-savings income and £11,200 is savings income.

Her net income is less than £43,001 so she is a basic rate taxpayer. She is therefore entitled to a personal savings allowance of £1,000.

Her non-savings income will use up all of the starting rate band and some of the basic rate band. She will therefore pay income tax on her savings income in excess of the personal savings allowance at 20%.

The income tax liability is:

	Income tax £
Non-savings income	
18,920 × 20%	3,784
Savings income	
1,000 × 0% (personal savings allowance)	0
10,200 × 20% (11,200 – 1,000)	2,040
30,120	
Income tax liability	5,824

This can be illustrated on the diagram as below.

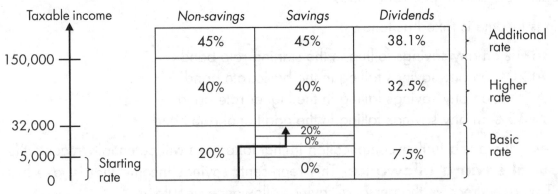

Illustration 4: Savings income example 2

Dave has net income of £90,000 (before the personal allowance) and taxable income of £79,000. Of this, £70,000 is non-savings income and £9,000 is savings income.

His net income is greater than £43,000 but less than £150,000 so he is a higher rate taxpayer. He is therefore entitled to a personal savings allowance of £500.

His non-savings income will use up all of the starting rate band and the basic rate band. He will therefore pay income tax on his savings income in excess of the personal savings allowance at 40%.

The income tax liability is:

	Income tax £
Non-savings income	
32,000 × 20%	6,400
38,000 × 40% (70,000 – 32,000) 70,000	15,200
Savings income	
500 × 0% (personal savings allowance)	0
8,500 × 40% (9,000 – 500) 79,000	3,400
Income tax liability	25,000

This can be illustrated on the diagram below.

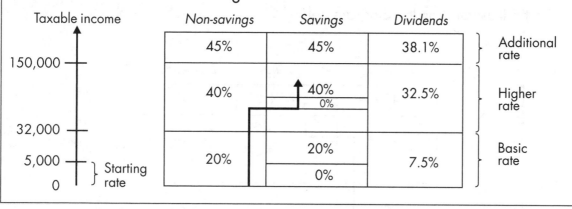

Illustration 5: Savings income example 3

Frank has net income of £180,000. He receives no personal allowance so his taxable income is also £180,000. Of this, £100,000 is non-savings income and £80,000 is savings income.

His net income is greater than £150,000 so he is an additional rate taxpayer. He is therefore not entitled to a personal savings allowance.

His non-savings income will use up all of the starting rate band and the basic rate band. He will therefore pay income tax on his savings income initially at 40% and then 45%.

The income tax liability is:

	Income tax £
Non-savings income	
32,000 × 20%	6,400
68,000 × 40% (100,000 – 32,000)	27,200
100,000	
Savings income	
50,000 × 40%	20,000
150,000	
30,000 × 45% (80,000 – 50,000)	13,500
£180,000	
Income tax liability	67,100

This can be illustrated on the diagram below.

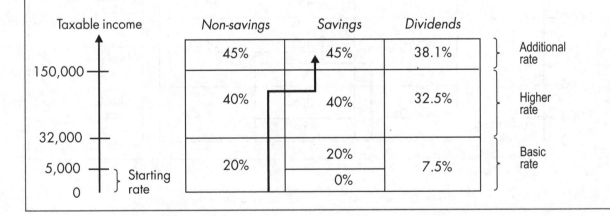

Activity 1: Income tax liability

In 2016/17 Jules, who is single, has employment income of £35,500 and building society interest of £9,000.

Required

Calculate the income tax liability.

Solution

	Non-savings income £	Savings income £	Total £

4 Savings income and the starting rate band

Remember that the order of taxation is:

(1) Non-savings income
(2) Savings income
(3) Dividend income

There is a special rate that applies to taxpayers who have no or low amounts of non-savings income but have savings income.

If any savings income falls within the first £5,000 of taxable income, then it is taxed at a special rate of 0%.

The personal savings allowance would also be available in these circumstances. Note that here it acts in addition to the starting rate band.

Illustration 6: Savings income starting rate

Tamara has net income in 2016/17 of £21,000 giving taxable income of £10,000 following the deduction of the personal allowance. £2,000 is non-savings income and £8,000 is savings income. As her net income is below £43,000 she is entitled to the full personal savings allowance of £1,000.

Her income tax liability is:

	Income tax £
Non-savings income	
2,000 × 20%	400
Savings income	
3,000 × 0%	0
5,000 (starting rate band limit)	
1,000 × 0% (personal savings allowance)	0
4,000 × 20% (8,000 – 3,000 – 1,000)	800
Income tax liability	1,200

This can be illustrated on the diagram below.

Calculation of tax liability

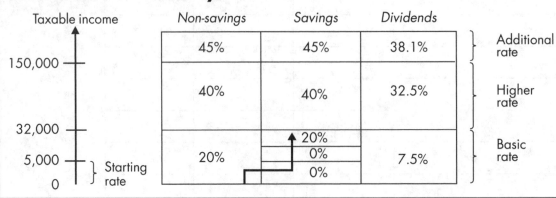

Activity 2: Starting rate band

Tegan earns a salary of £12,000. She receives bank interest of £40,000.

Required

Calculate her income tax liability for 2016/17.

Solution

	Non-savings income £	Savings income £	Total £

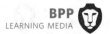

5 Dividend income

Once we have taxed non-savings income and savings income, we then move on to tax dividend income.

As before, we begin taxing dividend income in the bands at the point where we finished taxing the savings income.

Dividend income is taxed as follows:

- At 7.5% on any dividend income falling in the basic rate band

- At 32.5% on any dividend income falling in the higher rate band

- At 38.1% on any dividend income falling in the additional rate band

However, there is a further complication in that taxpayers will receive the dividend allowance. This represents dividend income that is taxed at 0%. All taxpayers receive a dividend allowance of £5,000 regardless of their level of net income.

Illustration 7: Dividend income

Douglas has taxable income of £165,000. Of this, £120,000 is non-savings income, £20,000 is savings income and £25,000 is dividend income.

Douglas is clearly an additional rate taxpayer so he will not receive a personal savings allowance. However, he is entitled to the dividend allowance.

The non-savings income of £120,000 uses all the basic rate band of £32,000 and £88,000 of the higher rate band. The £20,000 interest uses a further £20,000 of the higher rate band, leaving a balance of £10,000 remaining. The first £5,000 of dividend income is taxed at 0% because of the dividend allowance but this uses up £5,000 of the remaining higher rate band, leaving £5,000 available for the dividend. The next £5,000 of dividend is therefore taxed in the higher rate band at 32.5%, with the balance of £15,000 taxed at 38.1%.

The income tax liability is:

	Income tax £
Non-savings income	
32,000 × 20%	6,400
88,000 × 40%	35,200
Savings income	
20,000 × 40%	8,000
Dividend income	
5,000 × 0% (dividend allowance)	0
5,000 × 32.5%	1,625
150,000	
15,000 × 38.1% (25,000 – 5,000 – 5,000)	5,715
165,000	
Income tax liability	56,940

This can be illustrated on the diagram below.

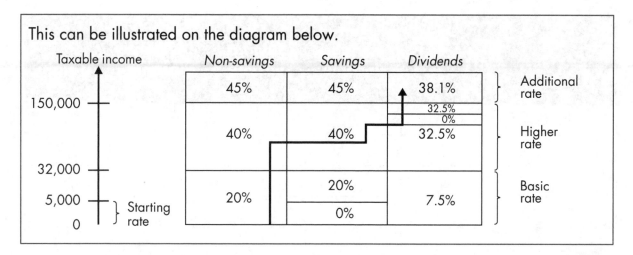

Activity 3: Income tax payable

Arthur has a salary of £125,000 (PAYE £42,000). He received bank interest of £10,000 and dividends of £10,000.

Required

Calculate the net income tax payable for 2016/17.

Solution

	Non-savings income £	Savings income £	Dividend income £	Total £

	Non-savings income £	Savings income £	Dividend income £	Total £

6 Extending the bands

Certain donations to UK registered charities or payments into personal pension schemes are eligible for tax relief.

Essentially, the income the taxpayer puts into the pension scheme/gives to charity is not taxable. The taxpayer therefore saves the tax they would have paid on that income.

Different taxpayers will therefore be entitled to relief at different rates.

Most taxpayers are employees who have already paid their tax via PAYE. By giving money to charity/paying into a pension they are therefore entitled to a refund of tax already paid on this income. Most taxpayers pay tax at 20% so making a payment of £100 would entitle them to a repayment of £20.

It would be onerous for the taxpayer and the Government if everyone who made such a payment had to apply to the Government for a tax refund so to simplify the administration payments are always made **net** of basic rate (20%) tax. The

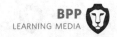

charity/pension will then reclaim the 20% tax from HMRC on behalf of all its donors in one go, saving much time and effort.

The taxpayer has therefore obtained relief at 20% as the charity/pension receives the full 100% but it has only cost the taxpayer 80%. This is effectively the same as the taxpayer giving the charity/pension 100% and then claiming the 20% tax back from the Government that they have already paid on that income.

If the taxpayer does pay tax at 20% then no further action is required on their part.

Higher rate (40%) taxpayers are entitled to an additional 20% (40% – 20%) relief on their gross donation/pension contribution. Additional rate taxpayers are entitled to an additional 25% (45% – 20%) relief on their gross donation/pension contribution.

Additional (20% or 25%) relief is given for charitable donations/pension contributions made by higher/additional rate taxpayers by a process known as 'extending the bands'. This moves income that would have been taxed at a higher rate into a lower rate band, effectively giving the taxpayer a discount on their tax bill.

The basic rate upper limit becomes:

32,000 + (payments × $^{100}/_{80}$) – income is moved out of higher rate into basic rate saving 20% (40% – 20%)

The higher rate limit becomes:

150,000 + (payment × $^{100}/_{80}$) – income is moved out of additional rate into higher rate saving a further 5% (45% – 40%). This combined with the basic rate extension above gives the taxpayer a 25% saving (20% + 5%).

Assessment focus point

If a taxpayer makes a payment to charity under Gift Aid or makes a payment into a personal pension scheme, gross up the amount paid by 100/80 and then add this total to the basic rate and higher rate band before calculating the tax liability.

Double check that the figure has not been given to you gross in the question. If it is already gross don't gross it up again.

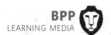

Illustration 8: Gift Aid donation

Gustav has taxable income (all non-savings) of £50,000 in 2016/17.

Assuming that Gustav does not make any Gift Aid donations or personal pension contributions in 2016/17 his income tax liability will be:

	£
32,000 × 20%	6,400
18,000 × 40%	7,200
50,000	13,600

Now think about the situation where Gustav makes a Gift Aid donation of £8,000 in 2016/17. The Gift Aid donation will have been paid net of 20% tax. This means that the gross amount of the payment is £8,000 × 100/80 = £10,000 and Gustav's basic rate band must be extended by £10,000. His income tax liability is calculated as follows:

	£
32,000 × 20%	6,400
10,000 (extended basic rate band) × 20%	2,000
8,000 × 40%	3,200
50,000	11,600

Extending the basic rate band means that £10,000 more income is taxed at the basic rate and therefore £10,000 less income is taxed at the higher rate. The difference between the tax liabilities with and without the Gift Aid donation is £10,000 × (40 − 20)% = £2,000. The total tax relief is:

	£
Basic rate relief given by net payment (10,000 − 8,000)	2,000
Higher rate relief given by extending basic rate band	2,000
Total tax relief (which equates to 40% of the gross donation)	4,000

Activity 4: Tax liability with Gift Aid donation

In 2016/17, Charlie has employment income of £100,000. He wishes to make a donation of £8,000 (net) to charity.

Required

For 2016/17, calculate Charlie's:

(a) **Taxable income**

£ [   ]

(b) **Tax liability if he does not make the donation**

£ [   ]

(c) Tax liability if he does make the donation

£ [   ]

(d) Total tax saved if he does make the donation

£ [   ]

Remember that a personal pension contribution or Gift Aid payment is deducted from total income before restricting the personal allowance. It is the **gross** payment that is deducted (payment × $^{100}/_{80}$).

7 Payroll giving and occupational pension schemes

A taxpayer may also donate to charity via their employer. Under payroll giving, the taxpayer requests that their employer pay some of their salary directly to charity.

A taxpayer may contribute to an occupational pension scheme. This is a pension scheme provided by the employer. Contributions will be deducted directly from the employee's salary.

The taxpayer will obtain tax relief on both of these payments. As they are deducted from salary, they reduce the taxpayer's taxable income and thus their tax liability.

Taxpayers will save at either 20%, 40% or 45% depending on their level of income.

There is no need to extend the basic rate band for these payments.

8 Tax planning

We have seen in previous chapters how income bearing assets may be transferred from one taxpayer to another to reduce the overall tax liability. We now see a further tax planning opportunity:

Even if both taxpayers pay tax at the same rate they should consider transferring assets between each other to ensure they get the maximum benefit from the savings allowance and the dividend allowance. For example if each party is paying tax at higher rate they will each receive a personal savings allowance of £500. If one party owns all the invested cash and is in receipt of £1,000 of interest then £500 of it will be above the allowance and will be taxable. If half of the cash is transferred to the other party then they will both be in receipt of £500 which will be covered by their personal savings allowance and together they will not pay tax.

People should also consider making charitable payments or payments into pensions to reduce their tax liability or to preserve the higher personal savings allowance. Again, with couples it makes more sense for the taxpayer paying tax at the higher rate to make the payment.

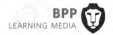

Chapter summary

- Income is categorised into different types: non-savings, savings and dividend. Each type of income suffers different rates of tax, depending on whether the income falls into the basic or higher rate bands or over the additional rate threshold.

- Non-savings income is taxed first (at 20%, then 40%, then 45%) then savings income (at 0%, then 20%, then 40%, then 45%) and finally dividend income (at 7.5%, then 32.5%, then 38.1%).

- The savings income starting rate of 0% applies to savings income within the savings income starting rate band.

- A personal savings allowance is available at £1,000 for a basic rate taxpayer, £500 for a higher rate taxpayer and £0 for an additional rate taxpayer. Savings income falling into the allowance is taxed at 0%. The allowance is added to the starting rate band but reduces the basic rate and higher rate band.

- A dividend allowance of £5,000 is available to all taxpayers. Dividends falling into this band are taxed at 0%. The allowance reduces the basic rate and higher rate bands.

- Gift Aid donations and personal pension contributions are paid net of basic rate (20%) tax.

- Extend the basic rate band by the gross amount of any Gift Aid donations and/or personal pension contributions paid by the taxpayer. This gives further tax relief to higher and additional rate taxpayers.

- Payments made to charity via payroll deduction or pension contributions made to an occupational scheme are simply deducted from salary.

- Tax deducted under the PAYE system is deducted in computing tax payable and can be repaid if it is greater than the taxpayer's liability.

BPP
LEARNING MEDIA

Keywords

- **Additional rate band:** income in excess of £150,000 is taxed here

- **Basic rate band:** the first £32,000 of income. The basic rate band may be extended by the gross amount of any Gift Aid donations and personal pension contributions paid by the taxpayer

- **Dividend allowance:** an amount of savings income that is taxed at 0%. This is £5,000 for all taxpayers

- **Higher rate band:** the next £118,000 of income. The upper limit to the higher rate band may be extended by the gross amount of any Gift Aid donations and personal pension contributions paid

- **Personal savings allowance:** an amount of savings income that is taxed at 0%. The amount varies depending on levels of income

- **Savings income starting rate band:** applies if the taxpayer has non-savings income of less than this amount and also has savings income

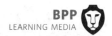

Activity 1: Income tax liability

	Non-savings income £	Savings income £	Total £
Employment income	35,500		35,500
Building society interest		9,000	9,000
Net income	35,500	9,000	44,500
Personal allowance	(11,000)		
Taxable income	24,500	9,000	33,500

Net income > 43,000 < £150,001 therefore £500 personal savings allowance available

	£
Non-savings income	
24,500 × 20%	4,900
Savings income	
500 × 0% (personal savings allowance)	0
7,000 × 20%	1,400
32,000	
1,500 (9,000 – 500 – 7,000) × 40%	600
Tax liability	6,900

Activity 2: Starting rate band

	Non-savings income £	Savings income £	Total £
Employment income	12,000		12,000
Bank interest		40,000	40,000
Net income	12,000	40,000	52,000
Less personal allowance	(11,000)		(11,000)
Taxable income	1,000	40,000	41,000

Net income > 42,000, < 150,000 so personal savings allowance of £500 available

		£
Non-savings income		
1,000 x 20%		200
Savings income		
4,000 × 0%		0
5,000		
500 × 0% (personal savings allowance)		0
26,500 × 20%		5,300
32,000		
9,000 × 40% (40,000 – 4,000 – 500 – 26,500)		3,600
Tax liability		9,100

Activity 3: Income tax payable

	Non-savings income £	Savings income £	Dividend income £	Total £
Employment income	125,000			125,000
Bank interest		10,000		10,000
Dividends			10,000	10,000
Net income	125,000	10,000	10,000	145,000
Personal allowance	(Nil)			(Nil)
Taxable income	125,000	10,000	10,000	145,000

Note. Total income is in excess of £122,000, so Arthur is not entitled to a personal allowance. Net income is greater than £43,000 but less than £150,000 so £500 savings allowance is available. Dividend allowance is always available.

	£
Non-savings income:	
32,000 × 20%	6,400
93,000 × 40%	37,200
125,000	
Savings income:	
500 × 0% (savings allowance)	0
9,500 × 40%	3,800
10,000	
Dividend income:	
5,000 × 0%	0
5,000 × 32.5%	1,625
10,000	
Tax liability	49,025
Less PAYE	(42,000)
Tax payable	7,025

Activity 4: Tax liability with Gift Aid donation

(a) Taxable income

£ | 89,000

Workings

Taxable income

	Non-savings income £
Employment income	100,000
Less personal allowance (income ≤ 100,000 ∴ no restriction)	(11,000)
Taxable income	89,000

(b) Tax liability if he does not make the donation

£ | 29,200

Workings

Tax liability without the donation

	£
32,000 × 20%	6,400
57,000 × 40%	22,800
89,000	
Tax liability	29,200

(c) Tax liability if he does make the donation

£ | 27,200

Workings

Tax liability with the donation

	£
Gross donation is $8,000 \times \dfrac{100}{80}$	10,000
Basic rate extends to 10,000 + 32,000	42,000
42,000 × 20%	8,400
47,000 × 40%	18,800
89,000	
	27,200

(d) Tax saved if he does make the donation

£ | 4,000 |

Workings

Tax saving (29,200 – 27,200)	= extra 2,000
which is 20% of the gross donation	
(8,000 × 100/80 = 10,000 @ 20%)	
Total relief:	
Obtained at source: 10,000 – 8,000	2,000
Reduction in tax liability (above)	2,000
Total	4,000
ie 40% of gross donation of 10,000	

Test your learning

1 At what rates is income tax charged on non-savings income?

Tick ONE box.

	✓
0%, 20%, 40% and 45%	
40% and 45%	
20% only	
20%, 40% and 45%	

2 In 2016/17 Albert has a salary of £16,600, £2,000 of building society interest and £3,000 of dividends.

Albert's income tax liability is:

£ [   ]

3 In 2016/17 Carol has a salary of £5,000, and has received building society interest of £18,000 and a dividend of £22,000.

Carol's income tax liability is:

£ [   ]

4 In 2016/17 Harry has a salary of £140,000, and has received building society interest of £20,000 and dividends of £30,000.

Harry's income tax liability is:

£ [   ]

5 **Explain how tax relief is given on Gift Aid donations.**

6 Doreen has the following sources of income in 2016/17.

	£
Gross pension income (tax deducted under PAYE £2,010)	17,000
Property income	3,500
Interest received from government stock	380
Dividends received	700
Premium bond prize	100

Calculate Doreen's income tax payable for the year.

7   Sase has the following income and outgoings in 2016/17.

	£
Business profits	36,600
Building society interest received	2,000
Dividends received	8,000
Gift Aid donation paid	1,600

Compute Sase's income tax payable for the year.

8   Vince is a higher rate taxpayer and makes a Gift Aid donation of £15,000 in 2016/17.

What is Vince's basic rate band in 2016/17?

Tick ONE Box.

	✓
£32,000	
£47,000	
£50,750	
£57,000	

Chargeable gains

8

Learning outcomes

1	**Analyse the theories, principles and rules that underpin taxation systems**
1.4	**Discuss residence and domicile** • The definitions of residence and domicile • The impact that each of these has on the taxation position of a UK taxpayer
4	**Account for capital gains tax**
4.1	**Discuss chargeable and exempt capital transactions** • Chargeable and exempt assets • Chargeable and exempt persons • Connected persons
4.2	**Calculate chargeable gains and allowable losses** • Calculate chargeable gains and allowable losses on normal capital disposals • Apply part disposals rules • Apply chattels and wasting chattel rules • Determine principal private residence relief
4.4	**Calculate capital gains tax payable** • Apply current exemptions • Treat capital losses • Apply rates of capital gains tax • Identify the date on which capital gains tax is due

Assessment context

Task 9 of the initial AAT sample assessment required the calculation of chargeable gains for a number of different disposals testing a variety of the different rules in this chapter including those for chattels, exempt assets and connected parties, 12 marks were available. Task 11 required you to calculate the capital gains tax payable for a number of different taxpayers in different circumstances.

Qualification context

You will not see the information in this chapter outside of this unit unless you are also studying *Business Tax*.

Business context

People sell assets for a variety of reasons. It is important to realise when a charge to capital gains tax arises and when capital gains tax needs to be paid if a taxpayer is to avoid paying interest and penalties.

Chapter overview

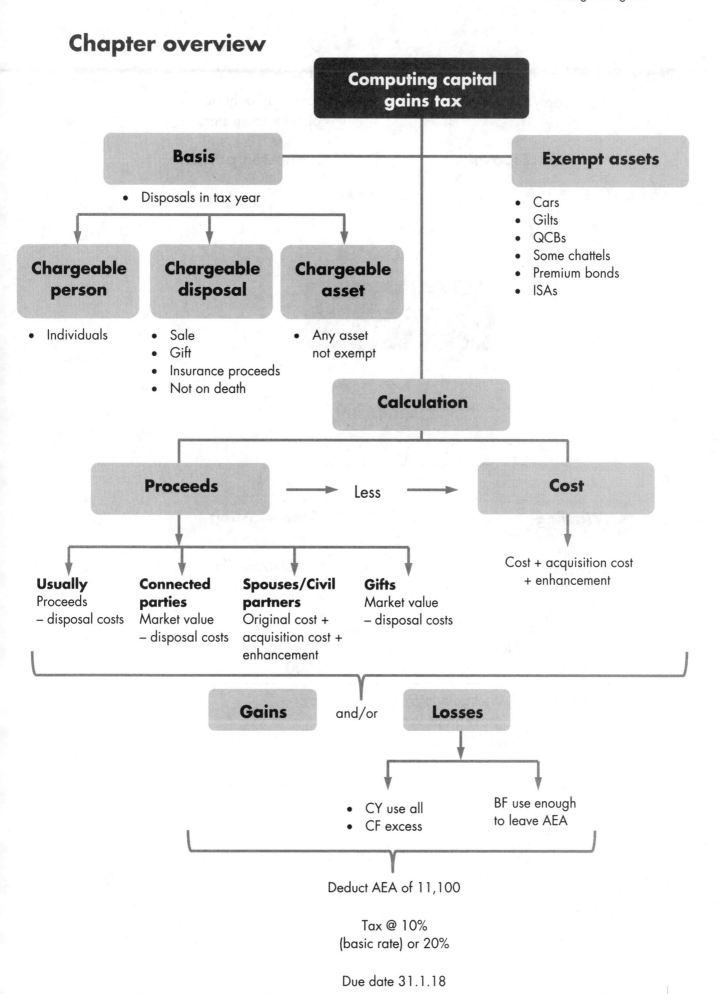

Computing capital gains tax

Basis
- Disposals in tax year

Exempt assets
- Cars
- Gilts
- QCBs
- Some chattels
- Premium bonds
- ISAs

Chargeable person
- Individuals

Chargeable disposal
- Sale
- Gift
- Insurance proceeds
- Not on death

Chargeable asset
- Any asset not exempt

Calculation

Proceeds → Less → **Cost**

Cost + acquisition cost + enhancement

Usually
Proceeds – disposal costs

Connected parties
Market value – disposal costs

Spouses/Civil partners
Original cost + acquisition cost + enhancement

Gifts
Market value – disposal costs

Gains and/or **Losses**

- CY use all
- CF excess

BF use enough to leave AEA

Deduct AEA of 11,100

Tax @ 10% (basic rate) or 20%

Due date 31.1.18

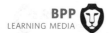

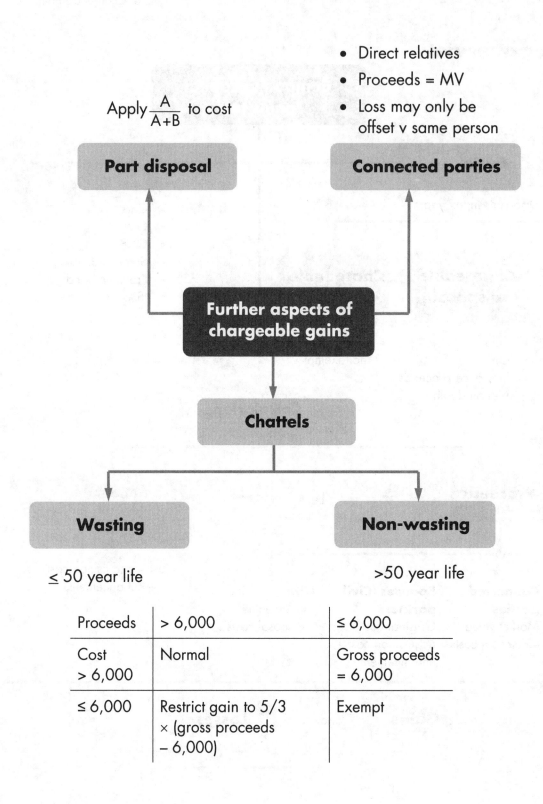

Apply $\dfrac{A}{A+B}$ to cost

Part disposal

- Direct relatives
- Proceeds = MV
- Loss may only be offset v same person

Connected parties

Further aspects of chargeable gains

Chattels

Wasting

≤ 50 year life

Non-wasting

>50 year life

Proceeds	> 6,000	≤ 6,000
Cost > 6,000	Normal	Gross proceeds = 6,000
≤ 6,000	Restrict gain to 5/3 × (gross proceeds – 6,000)	Exempt

Introduction

Income is a regular receipt that is expected to recur. A gain is a one-off disposal of a capital item.

Individuals pay **income tax** on income and **capital gains tax** on capital gains.

1 When does a chargeable gain arise?

For a disposable to be taxable there must be a **chargeable disposal** of a **chargeable asset** by a **chargeable person**.

1.1 Chargeable person

Individuals are chargeable persons.

1.2 Chargeable disposal

An individual is taxed on gains arising from disposals in the current tax year.

The following are the most important **chargeable disposals**:

- Sales of assets or parts of assets
- Gifts of assets or parts of assets
- The loss or destruction of an asset

A chargeable disposal occurs on the date of the contract (where there is one, whether written or oral), or the date of a conditional contract becoming unconditional.

Exempt disposals include:

- Transfers on death
- Gifts to charities

On death the heirs inherit assets as if they bought them at death for their then market values. There is no capital gain or allowable loss on death.

1.3 Chargeable assets

All assets are chargeable unless they are classified as exempt. The following are exempt:

- Motor vehicles suitable for private use
- UK government stocks (gilt-edged securities)
- Qualifying corporate bonds (company loan stock)
- **Wasting chattels** (greyhounds, racehorses) (see later)
- Premium bonds
- Investments held in an ISA

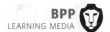

2 Calculation of chargeable gains and allowable losses

Illustration 1: Basic capital gains computation

Disposal consideration (or market value)	X
Less incidental costs of disposal	(X)
Net proceeds	X
Less allowable cost (including acquisition cost)	(X)
Less enhancement expenditure	(X)
Capital gain / (capital loss)	X/(X)

We now look at each of the items in the above proforma in turn.

2.1 Disposal consideration

Usually this is proceeds received. Note, though, that a disposal is deemed to take place at market value when the disposal is:

- A gift
- Made for a consideration that cannot be valued
- Deliberately sold for a consideration of less than market value
- Made to a connected person (see later)

Note that if a taxpayer makes a sale to an unconnected person and strikes a bad bargain then the actual proceeds achieved will be used. Market value is only used for a sale between unconnected persons when the taxpayer deliberately chooses to sell at undervalue to give the buyer a benefit.

2.2 Costs

The following costs are deducted in the above proforma:

(a) **Incidental costs of disposal**

These are the costs of selling an asset. They may include advertising costs, estate agents' fees, legal costs and valuation fees. These costs should be deducted separately from any other allowable costs.

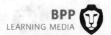

(b) **Allowable costs**

These include:

(i) The original purchase price of the asset

(ii) Costs incurred in purchasing the asset (estate agents' fees, legal fees, etc)

(c) **Enhancement expenditure**

This is capital expenditure which enhances the value of the asset and is reflected in the state or nature of the asset at the time of disposal.

Illustration 2: Calculation of capital gain

Jack bought a holiday cottage for £25,000. He paid legal costs of £600 on the purchase.

Jack spent £8,000 building an extension to the cottage.

Jack sold the cottage for £60,000. He paid estate agents' fees of £1,200 and legal costs of £750.

Jack's gain on sale is:

£	24,450

	£
Disposal consideration	60,000
Less incidental costs of disposal (1,200 + 750)	(1,950)
Net proceeds	58,050
Less allowable costs (25,000 + 600)	(25,600)
Less enhancement expenditure	(8,000)
Chargeable gain	24,450

Activity 1: Capital gain calculation

Mr Dunstable bought an asset for £15,000 in February 1986. He incurred legal fees of £500. He sold the asset for £38,500 incurring expenses of £1,500. While he owned the asset he improved it at a cost of £3,000.

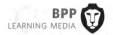

Required

Complete the table showing Mr Dunstable's gain.

Solution

	£
Proceeds	
Less selling expenses	_____
Net proceeds	
Less cost	
Less legal fees on purchase	
Less enhancement	_____
Capital gain	=====

3 Computing taxable gains in a tax year

An individual pays capital gains tax (CGT) on any **taxable gains** arising in a **tax year** (6 April to 5 April).

All the chargeable gains made in the tax year are added together, and any capital losses made in the same tax year are deducted to give net gains (or losses) for the year. Next we deduct any unrelieved capital losses brought forward from previous years. Finally the annual exempt amount is deducted to arrive at taxable gains, on which CGT will be applied.

Illustration 3: Year-end computation

	£
Current gains	X
Current losses (all)	(X)
Net gains	X
Losses b/fwd from earlier years (restricted)	(X)
Net capital gains	X
Annual exempt amount	(11,100)
Taxable gains	X

Unused annual exempt amounts cannot be carried forward.

3.1 Annual exempt amount

Key term

Annual exempt amount	This is the amount of capital gains a taxpayer may realise in a tax year before they have to pay capital gains tax.
	For 2016/17 it is £11,100.
	It is also known as the annual exemption.

All individuals are entitled to an annual exempt amount. As you can see above, it is the last deduction to be made in computing taxable gains, and effectively means that for 2016/17 the first £11,100 of chargeable gains is tax free for an individual.

3.2 Losses

If losses have been made in the current year they must be offset against the gains of that year even if this means that some or all of the annual exempt amount is wasted.

If the losses in a year are greater than the gains then the excess losses are carried forward.

When a capital loss is carried forward it is set against net gains in the next tax year but only to reduce the net gains in the next tax year down to the level of the annual exempt amount. This means the taxpayer does not lose the benefit of the annual exempt amount.

Any further loss remaining is carried forward.

Illustration 4: Capital losses

(a) Tim has chargeable gains for 2016/17 of £25,000 and allowable losses of £16,000. As the losses are current year losses they must be fully relieved against the gains to produce net gains of £9,000, despite the fact that net gains are below the annual exempt amount.

	£
Chargeable gains in tax year	25,000
Less losses in tax year	(16,000)
Net chargeable gains	9,000
Less annual exempt amount	(11,100)
Taxable gain	0

(b) Hattie has gains of £11,600 for 2016/17 and allowable losses brought forward of £6,000. Hattie restricts her loss relief to £500 so as to leave net gains of (£11,600 – £500) = £11,100, which will be exactly covered by the annual exempt amount for 2016/17.

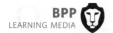

	£
Net chargeable gains	11,600
Less losses brought forward	(500)
Less annual exempt amount	(11,100)
Taxable gain	0

The remaining £5,500 of losses will be carried forward to 2017/18.

Activity 2: Current year losses

In 2016/17, Ted makes gains of £45,000 and £10,000. He also makes a loss of £48,000. Ted has no losses to bring forward from earlier years.

Required

Complete the following sentences:

Ted's net capital gain for 2016/17 before the annual exempt amount

is £ [   ]

Ted has a loss to carry forward of £ [   ]

Activity 3: Prior year losses

Tara makes a gain on a property in 2016/17 of £12,000 (proceeds of £25,000 less cost of £13,000). She makes no other disposals in the tax year. Tara has losses brought forward from the previous year of £10,000.

Required

Complete the following sentences:

Tara's net capital gain for 2016/17 before the annual exempt amount

is £ [   ]

Tara has a loss to carry forward of £ [   ]

4 Computing capital gains tax (CGT) payable

An individual's taxable gains are chargeable to CGT at the rate of 10% or 20% depending on the individual's taxable income for 2016/17.

If the individual is a basic rate taxpayer, then CGT is payable at 10% on an amount of taxable gains up to the amount of the taxpayer's **unused** basic rate band and at 20% on the excess.

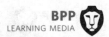

If the individual is a higher or additional rate taxpayer, then CGT is payable at 20% on all their taxable gains. Note the basic rate band covers taxable income and gains up to £32,000 (for 2016/17).

Note that a large gain may take a taxpayer out of the basic rate band and into the higher rate band. Don't forget that the bands will be extended by Gift Aid and/or personal pension scheme contributions.

Illustration 5: Calculating capital gains tax

(a) Sally has taxable income (ie the amount after the deduction of the personal allowance) of £10,000 in 2016/17 and made taxable gains (ie gains after deduction of the annual exempt amount) of £20,000 in 2016/17.

Sally's CGT liability is:

£20,000 × 10%	£2,000

The taxable income uses £10,000 of the basic rate band, leaving £22,000 of the basic rate band unused, therefore all of the taxable gain is taxed at 10%.

(b) Hector has taxable income of £50,000 in 2016/17 (ie he is a higher rate taxpayer). He made taxable gains of £10,000 in 2016/17.

Hector's CGT liability is:

£10,000 × 20%	£2,000

All of Hector's basic rate band has been taken up by the taxable income, therefore the taxable gain is taxed at 20%.

(c) Isabel has taxable income of £30,000 in 2016/17 and made taxable gains of £25,000 in 2016/17.

Isabel has (£32,000 − £30,000) = £2,000 of her basic rate band unused. Isabel's CGT liability is:

	£
2,000 × 10%	200
23,000 × 20%	4,600
25,000	4,800

Activity 4: Computing capital gains tax payable

Mr Dunstable (see Activity 1) had a chargeable gain of £18,500 in 2016/17. He has taxable income of £31,000.

Required

What is Mr Dunstable's capital gains tax payable?

£ [   ]

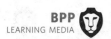

5 Self-assessment for CGT

5.1 Administration

CGT is payable on 31 January following the end of the tax year.

Unlike income tax there are no requirements for payments on account.

6 Special rules applying to specific disposals

Assessment focus point

The following rules need to be used in particular circumstances. Make sure you spot them in the assessment and apply them when required.

6.1 Part disposals and chattels

6.1.1 Part disposals

Sometimes part, rather than the whole, of an asset is disposed of. For instance, one-third of a piece of land may be sold. In this case, we need to be able to compute the chargeable gain or allowable loss arising on the part of the asset disposed of.

The problem is that, although we know what the disposal proceeds are for the part of the asset disposed of, we do not usually know what proportion of the 'cost' of the whole asset relates to that part. The solution to this is to **use the following fraction to determine the cost of the part disposed of**.

Formula to learn

The fraction is:

$$\frac{A}{A+B} = \frac{\text{Value of the part disposed of}}{\text{Value of the part disposed of} + \text{Market value of the remainder}}$$

A is the 'gross' proceeds (or market value) before deducting incidental costs of disposal.

B is the market value of the part of the asset that was not sold.

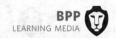

Illustration 6: Part disposal calculation

	£
Gross proceeds	X
Less selling costs	(X)
	X
Less:	
Original cost of the whole asset $\times \dfrac{A}{A+B}$	(C)
Gain	X

Illustration 7: Part disposal

Mr Jones bought 4 acres of land for £270,000. He sold 1 acre of the land at auction for £200,000, before auction expenses of 15%. The market value of the 3 remaining acres is £460,000.

The cost of the land being sold is:

$$\frac{200,000}{200,000 + 460,000} \times £270,000 = £81,818$$

	£
Disposal proceeds	200,000
Less incidental costs of sale (15% × £200,000)	(30,000)
Net proceeds	170,000
Less cost (see above)	(81,818)
Chargeable gain	88,182

Activity 5: Part disposal

Tom bought 10 acres of land for £20,000.

He sold 3 acres of land for £10,000 incurring disposal costs of £950 when the remaining 7 acres were worth £36,000.

Required

Complete the following sentences:

The gain on the disposal of the land is £

The cost of the remaining land carried forward is £

6.1.2 Chattels

Chattels	are tangible moveable property.
Wasting chattel	is a chattel with an estimated remaining useful life of 50 years or less, eg a racehorse or greyhound.

Wasting chattels are exempt from CGT so there are no chargeable gains and no allowable losses.

Non-wasting chattels are chargeable to CGT in the normal way, subject to the following exceptions/restrictions.

Illustration 8: Rule for computing gains/losses on non-wasting chattels

≤ 6,000	≤ 6,000	Wholly exempt	• No need to calculate any gain
≤ 6,000	> 6,000	Any gain restricted to max of: $\frac{5}{3}$ (Gross proceeds – £6,000)	• Calculate gain, compare to the maximum, take the lower figure
> 6,000	≤ 6,000	Gross proceeds deemed to be £6,000	• Do normal calculation but always use £6,000 as gross proceeds figure
> 6,000	> 6,000	Wholly taxable	• Calculate a gain using the normal rules

Illustration 9: Proceeds > £6,000, Cost < £6,000

John purchased a painting for £3,000. On 1 January 2017 he sold the painting at auction.

If the gross sale proceeds are £4,000, the gain on sale will be exempt.

If the gross sale proceeds are £8,000 with costs of sale of 10%, the gain arising on the disposal of the painting will be calculated as follows:

	£
Gross proceeds	8,000
Less incidental costs of sale (10% × £8,000)	(800)
Net proceeds	7,200
Less cost	(3,000)
Chargeable gain	4,200
Gain cannot exceed 5/3 × £(8,000 – 6,000)	3,333

Therefore chargeable gain is £3,333.

Illustration 10: Proceeds < £6,000, Cost > £6,000

Magee purchased an antique desk for £8,000. She sold the desk in an auction for £4,750 net of auctioneer's fees of 5% in November 2016.

Magee obviously has a loss and therefore the allowable loss is calculated on deemed proceeds of £6,000. The costs of disposal can be deducted from the deemed proceeds of £6,000.

	£
Deemed disposal proceeds	6,000
Less incidental costs of disposal (£4,750 × 5/95)	(250)
	5,750
Less cost	(8,000)
Allowable loss	(2,250)

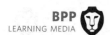

Activity 6: Chattels

(a) Orlando Gibbons purchased a rare manuscript for £500. He sold it several years later for £9,000, before deducting the auctioneer's commission of £1,000.

(b) He also had an antique bought for £7,000 which he sold 2 years later for £3,000.

Required

Complete the following sentences:

(a) The chargeable gain on the disposal is £ [   ]

(b) The loss on the disposal is £ [   ]

6.2 Transfers to connected persons

If a disposal by an individual is made to a connected person, **the disposal is deemed to take place at the market value of the asset**.

If an **allowable loss arises** on the disposal, it can **only be set against gains** arising in the same or future tax years from disposals **to the same connected person**, and the loss can only be set off if they are still connected with the person making the loss.

For this purpose an individual is connected with:

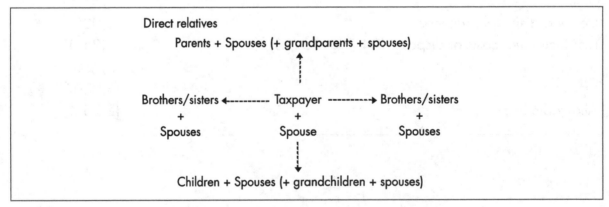

6.3 Transfers between spouses/civil partners

Spouses/civil partners are taxed as two separate people. Each individual has an annual exempt amount, and allowable losses of one individual cannot be set against gains of the other.

Disposals between spouses/civil partners do not give rise to chargeable gains or allowable losses. The disposal is said to be on a **'no gain/no loss'** basis. The acquiring spouse/civil partner takes the base cost of the disposing spouse/civil partner.

Activity 7: Transfers between spouses/civil partners

William sold an asset to his wife Kate in May 2015 for £32,000 when its market value was £45,000. William acquired the asset for £14,000 in June 2005.

Required

Calculate the chargeable gain on this transfer. Tick one box.

	✓
Nil	
£18,000	
£31,000	
£13,000	

7 Residence issues

Taxpayers who are resident and domiciled in the UK pay tax on all of their gains regardless as to where the assets are located.

Taxpayers who are resident but not domiciled in the UK will definitely pay tax on the disposal of assets located in the UK. Assets located overseas may be subject to the remittance basis. If this applies the taxpayer will only pay tax on the gain if the proceeds are brought back into the UK.

Non-resident taxpayers will not have to pay capital gains tax on any assets.

8 Tax planning

Consider:

- Delaying sale of an asset until after the end of the tax year, this would give you a whole extra year until you had to pay the tax and allow you to use next year's annual exempt amount (you may have already used this year's).

- Spouses and civil partners may transfer assets at no gain no loss. This effectively transfers the asset over at its original cost so that the gain will be the same whichever party sells it. It therefore makes sense to ensure an asset is sold by the spouse/civil partner who:

  - Pays tax at a lower rate
  - Has an unused annual exemption
  - Has capital losses

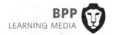

Chapter summary

- A chargeable gain arises when there is a chargeable disposal of a chargeable asset by a chargeable person.

- Enhancement expenditure can be deducted in computing a chargeable gain if it is reflected in the state and nature of the asset at the time of disposal.

- Taxable gains are net chargeable gains for a tax year (ie minus allowable losses of the current tax year and any unrelieved capital losses brought forward) minus the annual exempt amount.

- Losses brought forward can only reduce net chargeable gains down to the amount of the annual exempt amount.

- The rates of CGT are 10% and 20%, but the lower rate of 10% only applies if and to the extent that the individual has any unused basic rate band.

- CGT is payable by 31 January following the end of the tax year.

- There is a special page to complete for capital gains on the tax return.

- CGT is self-assessed and has the same rules about notification of chargeability, penalties and interest as income tax.

- On the part disposal of an asset the formula A/(A + B) must be applied to work out the cost attributable to the part disposed of.

- Wasting chattels are exempt assets (eg racehorses and greyhounds).

- If a non-wasting chattel is sold for gross proceeds of £6,000 or less and was bought for £6,000 or less then any gain arising is exempt.

- If gross proceeds exceed £6,000 on the sale of a non-wasting chattel but the cost is less than £6,000, any gain arising on the disposal of the asset is limited to 5/3 × (Gross proceeds − £6,000).

- If the gross proceeds are less than £6,000 on the sale of a non-wasting chattel but it was bought for more than £6,000 any loss otherwise arising is restricted by deeming the gross proceeds to be £6,000.

- A disposal to a connected person takes place at market value.

- For individuals, connected people are broadly brothers, sisters, lineal ancestors and descendants and their spouses/civil partners plus similar relations of a spouse/civil partner.

- Losses on disposals to connected people can only be set against gains on disposals to the same connected person.

- Disposals between spouses/civil partners take place on a no gain/no loss basis.

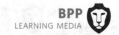

Keywords

- **Chargeable asset:** any asset that is not an exempt asset

- **Chargeable disposal:** a sale or gift of an asset

- **Chargeable person:** an individual or company

- **Chattel:** tangible moveable property

- **Connected person:** a close relation of the taxpayer or their spouse/civil partner

- **Enhancement expenditure:** capital expenditure that enhances the value of the asset and is reflected in the state or nature of the asset at the time of disposal

- **Exempt disposal:** a disposal on which no chargeable gain or allowable loss arises

- **Part disposal:** when part of an, rather than a whole, asset is disposed of

- **Taxable gains:** the chargeable gains of an individual for a tax year, after deducting allowable losses of the same tax year, any unrelieved capital losses brought forward and the annual exempt amount

- **Wasting chattel:** a chattel with an estimated remaining useful life of 50 years or less

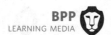

Activity 1: Capital gain calculation

	£
Proceeds	38,500
Less selling expenses	(1,500)
Net proceeds	37,000
Less cost	(15,000)
Less legal fees on purchase	(500)
Less enhancement	(3,000)
Capital gain	18,500

Activity 2: Current year losses

Ted's net capital gain for 2016/17 before the annual exempt amount is

£ | 7,000 |

Ted has a loss to carry forward of £ | nil |

Workings

	£
Gains 45,000 + 10,000	55,000
Less loss	(48,000)
Net capital gains	7,000
Less annual exempt amount	(11,100)
Taxable gains	Nil
The balance of the annual exempt amount is wasted.	

Activity 3: Prior year losses

Tara's net capital gain for 2016/17 before the annual exempt amount is

£ | 11,100 |

Tara has a loss to carry forward of £ | 9,100 |

Workings

	£
Gain of 2016/17	12,000
Less losses b/f (bal)	(900)
Net gain	11,100
Less annual exempt amount	(11,100)
Taxable gains	Nil
Losses to c/f £(10,000 – 900)	9,100

Activity 4: Computing capital gains tax payable

Mr Dunstable's capital gains tax payable is £ | 1,380 |

Workings

	£
Capital gain	18,500
Less annual exempt amount	(11,100)
Taxable gain	7,400
Basic rate band	32,000
Taxable income	(31,000)
Basic rate band remaining	1,000

	£
Capital gains tax payable	
1,000 × 10%	100
6,400 × 20%	1,280
7,400	1,380

Activity 5: Part disposal

The gain on the disposal of the land is £ | 4,702 |

The cost of the remaining land carried forward is £ | 15,652 |

Workings

	£
Gross proceeds	10,000
Less disposal costs	(950)
Net proceeds	9,050
Cost $\dfrac{10}{10+36} \times 20,000$	(4,348)
	4,702
Cost of remaining land for future CGT calculations: = 20,000 – 4,348	15,652

Activity 6: Chattels

(a)   The chargeable gain on the disposal is £ [5,000]

Workings

Non-wasting chattel: cost ≤ £6,000, proceeds > £6,000	£
Proceeds	9,000
Less commission	(1,000)
Net proceeds	8,000
Less cost	(500)
Capital gain	7,500
$\frac{5}{3}$ (Gross proceeds – 6,000)	
$= \frac{5}{3}$ (9,000 – 6,000)	
= 5,000	
∴ take lower gain 5,000	5,000

(b)   The loss on the disposal is £ [1,000]

Workings

Non-wasting chattel: cost > £6,000, proceeds ≤ £6,000	£
Proceeds (deemed)	6,000
Less cost	(7,000)
Allowable loss	(1,000)

Activity 7: transfers between spouses/civil partners

The chargeable gain on transfer is:

	✓
Nil	✓
£18,000	
£31,000	
£13,000	

The transfer takes place at no gain/no loss and Kate assumes the base cost of £14,000 as her cost.

Test your learning

1   **Tick to show if the following disposals would be chargeable or exempt for CGT.**

	Chargeable ✓	Exempt ✓
A gift of an antique necklace		
The sale of a building		
Sale of a racehorse		

2   Janet bought a plot of land in July 2006 for £80,000. She spent £10,000 on drainage in April 2009. She sold the land for £200,000 in August 2016.

Using the proforma layout provided, compute the gain on sale.

	£
Proceeds of sale	
Less cost	
Less enhancement expenditure	
Chargeable gain	

3   Philip has chargeable gains of £171,000 and allowable losses of £5,300 in 2016/17. Losses brought forward at 6 April 2016 amount to £10,000.

The amount liable to CGT in 2016/17 is:

£ _____

The losses carried forward are:

£ _____

4   Martha is a higher rate taxpayer who made chargeable gains (before the annual exempt amount) of £23,900 in October 2016.

Martha's CGT liability for 2016/17 is:

£ _____

5   **The payment date for capital gains tax for 2016/17 is (insert date XX/XX/XXXX):**

_____

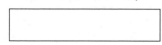

6   Richard sells 4 acres of land (out of a plot of 10 acres) for £38,000 in July 2016. Costs of disposal amount to £3,000. The 10-acre plot cost £41,500. The market value of the 6 acres remaining is £48,000.

The chargeable gain/allowable loss arising is:

Tick ONE box.

	✓
£16,663	
£17,500	
£19,663	
£18,337	

7   Mustafa bought a non-wasting chattel for £3,500.

The gain arising if he sells it for:

(a) £5,800 after deducting selling expenses of £180 is:

£ [   ]

(b) £8,200 after deducting selling expenses of £220 is:

£ [   ]

8   **Decide whether the following statement is true or false.**

A loss arising on a disposal to a connected person can be set against any gains arising in the same tax year or in subsequent tax years.

	✓
True	
False	

9   **Decide whether the following statement is true or false.**

No gain or loss arises on a disposal to a spouse/civil partner.

	✓
True	
False	

10 Complete the table by ticking the appropriate box for each scenario.

	Actual proceeds used	Deemed proceeds (market value) used	No gain or loss basis
Paul sells an asset to his civil partner Joe for £3,600.			
Grandmother gives an asset to her grandchild worth £1,000.			
Sarah sells an asset worth £20,000 to her best friend Cathy for £12,000. Sarah knows the asset is worth £20,000.			

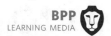

Share disposals

9

Learning outcomes

4	Account for capital gains tax
4.3	**Calculate gains and losses arising on the disposal of shares** • Apply matching rules for individuals • Account for bonus issues • Account for rights issues

Assessment context

Shares were tested for 10 marks in Task 10 of the initial AAT sample assessment. The task will be assessed by free data entry of all workings and will be human marked.

Qualification context

Share disposals by individuals also feature in *Business Tax*. You will not see these rules anywhere else in your qualification.

Business context

A tax practitioner needs to be able to calculate capital gains tax payable on the disposal of shares for their clients.

Chapter overview

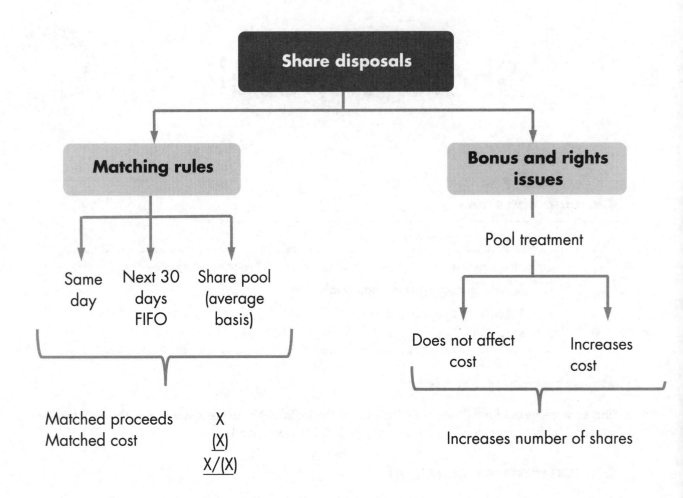

Share disposals

Matching rules

Same day

Next 30 days FIFO

Share pool (average basis)

Matched proceeds   X
Matched cost   (X)
           X/(X)

Bonus and rights issues

Pool treatment

Does not affect cost

Increases cost

Increases number of shares

Introduction

In this chapter we are going to look at special rules that apply when shares are sold.

1 Share disposal rules

1.1 Matching rules

Shares present special problems when computing gains or losses on disposal. For instance, suppose that a taxpayer buys some shares in X plc on the following dates:

	No of shares	Cost £
5 July 1992	150	195
17 January 1997	100	375
2 July 2016	100	1,000

On 15 June 2016, he sells 220 of his shares for £3,300. **To work out his chargeable gain, we need to be able to identify which shares** out of his three holdings **were actually sold**. Since one share is identical to any other, it is not possible to work this out by reference to factual evidence.

As a result, it has been necessary to devise 'matching rules'. These allow us to identify on a disposal which shares have been sold and so **work out what the allowable cost** (and therefore the gain) **on disposal should be**. These matching rules are considered in detail below.

Assessment focus point

It is very important that you understand the matching rules. These rules are very regularly assessed and if you do not understand them you will not be able to get any part of the task right.

Matching rules

Shares sold should be matched with purchases in the following order:

(1) Acquisitions on the same day as disposal.

(2) Acquisitions within the following 30 days on a first in, first out (FIFO) basis.

(3) Shares from the share pool. The share pool includes all other shares not acquired on the dates above, and is explained below.

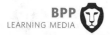

Illustration 1: Matching rules

Noah acquired shares in Ark Ltd as follows.

2 August 2012	10,000 shares
25 April 2014	10,000 shares
17 June 2016	1,000 shares
19 June 2016	2,000 shares

Noah sold 15,000 shares on 17 June 2016.

Which shares is he selling for capital gains tax purposes?

Noah will match his disposal of 15,000 shares on 17 June 2016 as follows:

(1) 1,000 shares bought on 17 June 2016 (same day)
(2) 2,000 shares bought on 19 June 2016 (next 30 days, FIFO basis)
(3) 12,000 shares from the 20,000 shares in the share pool

Illustration 2: Basic computation

	£	£
For each batch of matched shares:		
Proportion of proceeds	X	
Less cost (if from share pool W1)	(X)	
		X

(W1) Share pool

	No of shares	Cost £
Shares bought/sold	X	X

1.2 Share pool

The share pool includes shares acquired up to the day before the disposal on which we are calculating the gain or loss. It grows when an acquisition is made and shrinks when a disposal is made.

The calculation of the share pool value

To compute the value of the share pool, set up two columns of figures:

(a) The number of shares
(b) The cost of the shares

Each time shares are acquired, both the number and the cost of the acquired shares are added to those already in the pool.

When there is a disposal from the pool, both the number of shares being disposed of and a cost relating to those shares are deducted from the pool. The cost of the disposal is calculated as a proportion of total cost in the pool, based on the number of shares being sold.

Illustration 3: The share pool

Jackie bought 10,000 shares in X plc for £6,000 in August 1996 and another 10,000 shares for £9,000 in December 2008.

She sold 12,000 shares for £24,000 in August 2016.

The gain is:

	£
Proceeds of sale	24,000
Less allowable cost (W1)	(9,000)
Chargeable gain	15,000

(W1) The share pool is:

	No of shares	Cost £
August 1996 acquisition	10,000	6,000
December 2008 acquisition	10,000	9,000
	20,000	15,000
August 2016 disposal (£15,000 × 12,000/20,000 = £9,000)	(12,000)	(9,000)
c/f	8,000	6,000

Activity 1: Matching rules

Mr L made the following purchases of ordinary shares in H plc:

Date	Number	Cost
15 May 2002	2,200	8,800
1 May 2016	400	3,000
17 May 2016	500	4,500

On 1 May 2016 Mr L sold 1,600 shares for £14,000.

Required

What is the chargeable gain or loss for 2016/17 on the disposal of these shares? Clearly show the balance of shares to be carried forward.

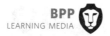

Solution

	Number	£

Activity 2: Share pool

Mr Lambert purchased the following holdings in Grande plc:

Date	Number	Cost £
January 1985	3,000	5,000
February 1987	1,000	4,000

In May 2016 he sold 2,000 shares for £14,000.

Required

What is the chargeable gain or loss for 2016/17 on the disposal of these shares? Clearly show the balance of shares to be carried forward.

Solution

	Number	£

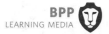

1.3 Bonus and rights issues

1.3.1 Bonus issues

Bonus issues are free shares given to existing shareholders in proportion to their existing shareholding. For example, a shareholder may own 2,000 shares. The company makes a 1 share for every 2 shares held bonus issue (called a 1 for 2 bonus issue). The shareholder will then have an extra 1,000 shares, giving them 3,000 shares overall.

Bonus shares are treated as being acquired at the date of the original acquisition of the underlying shares giving rise to the bonus issue.

Since bonus shares are issued at no cost there is **no need to adjust the original cost**.

1.3.2 Rights issues

In a **rights issue**, a **shareholder is offered the right to buy additional shares by the company in proportion to the shares already held**.

The difference between a bonus issue and a rights issue is that in a rights issue the new shares are paid for. This results in an **adjustment to the original cost**.

For matching purposes, bonus and rights shares are treated as if they were acquired on the same day as the shareholder's original holdings.

Illustration 4: Bonus and rights issues

Jonah acquired 20,000 shares for £34,200 in T plc in April 2005. There was a 1 for 2 bonus issue in May 2010 and a 1 for 5 rights issue in August 2015 at £1.20 per share.

Jonah sold 30,000 shares for £45,000 in December 2016.

The gain on sale is:

	£
Proceeds of sale	45,000
Less allowable cost (W1)	(34,500)
Chargeable gain	10,500

(W1) The share pool is constructed as follows:

	No of shares	Cost £
April 2005 acquisition	20,000	34,200
May 2010 bonus 1 for 2 (1/2 × 20,000 = 10,000)	10,000	–
	30,000	34,200
August 2015 rights 1 for 5 @ £1.20 (1/5 × 30,000 = 6,000 shares × £1.20 = £7,200)	6,000	7,200
	36,000	41,400
December 2016 disposal (£41,400 × 30,000/36,000 = £34,500)	(30,000)	(34,500)
c/f	6,000	6,900

Activity 3: Bonus and rights issues

Richard had the following transactions in S plc.

1.10.95	Bought 10,000 shares for £15,000
11.9.99	Bought 2,000 shares for £5,000
1.2.00	Took up rights issue 1 for 2 at £2.75 per share
5.9.05	2 for 1 bonus issue
14.10.16	Sold 15,000 shares for £15,000

Required

Calculate the gain or loss made on these shares. All workings must be shown in your calculations.

Solution

	Number	£

2 Tax planning

The tax planning ideas we considered in the previous chapter are still relevant here. One further matter to consider is that a holding of shares can be easily split so if a married couple/civil partnership were going to sell some shares and realise a large gain they could split the ownership between them before the sale. Instead of realising one gain they now have one gain each meaning that they could both use their annual exempt amounts rather than leaving one to go to waste (assuming they had no other disposals in the year).

Chapter summary

- The matching rules are:

  (1)   Same day acquisitions
  (2)   Next 30 days' acquisitions on a FIFO basis
  (3)   Shares in the share pool

- The share pool runs up to the day before disposal.

- Bonus issue and rights issue shares are acquired in proportion to the shareholder's existing holding.

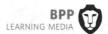

- **Bonus shares:** shares that are issued free to shareholders based on original holdings

- **Rights issues:** similar to bonus issues except that in a rights issue shares must be paid for

Activity answers

Activity 1: Matching rules

	Shares
Same day	400
Next 30 days	500
Share pool	700 ß
Disposal	1,600

(1) Match with same day

	£	£
Proceeds 400/1,600 × 14,000	3,500	
Cost	(3,000)	
		500

(2) Match with next 30 days

	£	£
Proceeds 500/1,600 × 14,000	4,375	
Cost	(4,500)	
		(125)

(3) Match with share pool

	£	£
Proceeds 700/1,600 × 14,000	6,125	
Cost (W)	(2,800)	
		3,325
Net gain		3,700

(W) Share pool

	Number	Cost
15.5.02	2,200	8,800
Disposal 700/2,200 × 8,800	(700)	(2,800)
	1,500	6,000

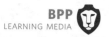

Activity 2: Share pool

Matching rules: The shares were all acquired prior to the date of disposal so they are all in the share pool.

	£
Proceeds	14,000
Cost (W1)	(4,500)
Gain	9,500

Share pool (W1)

	Number	Cost £
January 1985		
Purchase	3,000	5,000
February 1987		
Purchase	1,000	4,000
	4,000	9,000
May 2016		
Disposal 2,000/4,000 × 9,000	(2,000)	(4,500)
	2,000	4,500

Activity 3: Bonus and rights issues

Matching rules: All bought prior to date of disposal so all from share pool.

Gain

	£
Proceeds	15,000
Less cost (W1)	(10,139)
Gain	4,861

(W1) Share pool

	Number	Cost £
1.10.95	10,000	15,000
11.9.99 acquisition	2,000	5,000
	12,000	20,000
1.2.00 1:2 rights @ £2.75	6,000	16,500
	18,000	36,500
5.9.05 2:1 bonus	36,000	–
	54,000	36,500
14.10.16 sale 15,000/54,000 × 36,500	(15,000)	(10,139)
	39,000	26,361

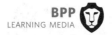

1   Tasha bought 10,000 shares in V plc in August 1994 for £5,000 and a further 10,000 shares for £16,000 in April 2009. She sold 15,000 shares for £30,000 in November 2016.

   Tick to show what her chargeable gain is.

   Tick ONE box.

	✓
£15,750	
£11,500	
£17,000	
£14,250	

2   **Tick to show whether the following statement is true or false.**

   In both a bonus issue and a rights issue, there is an adjustment to the original cost of the shares.

	✓
True	
False	

3   Marcus bought 2,000 shares in X plc in May 2003 for £12,000. There was a 1 for 2 rights issue at £7.50 per share in December 2004. Marcus sold 2,500 shares for £20,000 in March 2017.

   His chargeable gain is:

£	

4   Mildred bought 6,000 shares in George plc in June 2011 for £15,000. There was a 1 for 3 bonus issue in August 2012. Mildred sold 8,000 shares for £22,000 in December 2016.

   Her chargeable gain is:

£	

5   **What are the share matching rules?**

Principal private residence 10

Learning outcomes

Having studied this chapter, you will be able to:

4	**Account for capital gains tax**
4.2	**Calculate chargeable gains and allowable losses** • Determine principal private residence relief

Assessment context

This topic is included in the syllabus but was not tested in the initial AAT sample assessment.

Qualification context

You will not be tested on these rules outside of this unit.

Business context

Selling a house could trigger a substantial capital gains tax liability. A practitioner needs to be able to recognise when these rules apply to reduce or exempt the gain.

Chapter overview

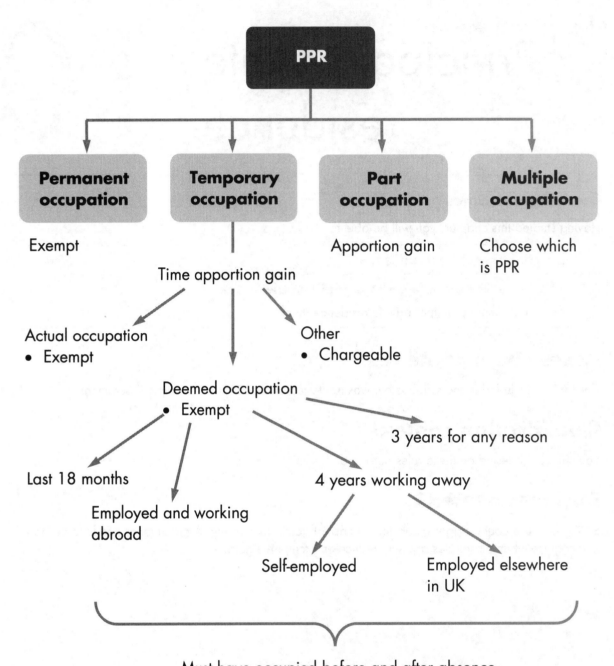

BPP
LEARNING MEDIA

Introduction

In this chapter we are going to look at special rules that apply when a taxpayer sells the property that they have lived in.

1 Principal private residence (PPR) relief

1.1 General rule

Key term

Principal private residence	This is an individual's only or main residence. It includes a garden of up to half a hectare. There is usually no capital gains tax liability when an individual sells their residence because of PPR relief.

If a taxpayer has lived in the residence **for the whole period of ownership** then there will be **no capital gain when the property is sold**. If the taxpayer has not lived there for the whole period of ownership than **only the gain relating to the period of occupation will be exempt**. This will be calculated by **time apportioning** the gain.

Likewise, if the property is sold at a loss then no capital loss may be claimed.

Formula to learn

Illustration – PPR relief is calculated as:

$$\text{Gain} \times \frac{\text{Period of occupation}}{\text{Period of ownership}}$$

1.2 Periods of occupation

Even though the taxpayer may not actually be occupying the property we may be able to treat it for tax purposes as if the taxpayer was actually in residence thus giving exemption from tax. These are what we call periods of **deemed occupation**.

Key term

Deemed occupation	A period of time when HMRC will treat the taxpayer as occupying the property for the purposes of claiming PPR relief even though they are not actually there.

The last 18 months are always deemed occupation in full, provided the property was the taxpayer's PPR at some point.

Certain periods of absence are deemed occupation, providing that they are preceded and followed (at any time whatsoever) by actual occupation:

Deemed occupation

- Any period during which the owner was abroad by reason of their employment

- Any periods (not exceeding four years in total) during which the employed owner was required to work away from home in the UK

- Any periods (not exceeding four years in total) during which the owner, if self-employed, was working away from home in the UK or overseas

- Any periods, for whatever reason, not exceeding three years in total

1.3 Part occupation

If any part of the residence is not occupied by the owner for residence purposes, PPR relief will be proportionately withdrawn. For example, if the garage was used as a workshop and one bedroom was used as a home office for a business, then the PPR would only be available on the percentage used for residential purposes.

If the property had been used for different purposes at different times then there would need to be an apportionment of relief based on time and use.

1.4 More than one residence

The taxpayer may choose which home is to be their PPR, provided that each has been occupied at some point.

If the owner is unable to occupy their own home because they are required to occupy job-related accommodation, their own home will be deemed to be their main residence, provided that they intend to occupy it at some point.

1.5 More than one occupier

Married couples/civil partners are only allowed one exemption between them.

Illustration 1: Principal private residence relief

Mr A purchased a house for £50,000 on 31 March 1997. He lived in the house until 30 June 1997. He was then sent to work abroad by his employer for 5 years before returning to the UK to live in the house again on 1 July 2002. He stayed in the house for 6 months before moving out to live with friends until the house was sold on 31 December 2016 for £150,000.

First work out the total period of ownership:

31 March 1997 to 31 December 2016 = 19 years and 9 months (or 237 months).

Next, decide what periods are chargeable and which are exempt:

		Exempt months	Chargeable months
(i)	1 April 1997 to 30 June 1997	3	–
(ii)	1 July 1997 to 30 June 2002	60	–
(iii)	1 July 2002 to 31 December 2002	6	–
(iv)	1 January 2003 to 30 June 2015	–	150
(v)	1 July 2015 to 31 December 2016	18	–
		87	150

Explanations:

(i)   **April 1997 to June 1997.** Actual occupation.

(ii) **July 1997 to June 2002.** Covered by the exemption for periods of absence during which the owner is required by his employment to live abroad. The period is both preceded and followed by a period of owner occupation.

(iii) **July 2002 to December 2002.** Actual occupation.

(iv) **January 2003 to June 2015.** This period is not eligible to be partly covered by the exemption for three years of absence for any reason, as it is not followed by a period of actual occupation.

(v)   **July 2015 to December 2016.** Covered by the final 18 months' exemption.

Then, calculate the chargeable gain after the exemption has been applied:

	£
Disposal proceeds	150,000
Less cost	(50,000)
Gain before PPR	100,000
Less exempt under PPR provisions	
$\dfrac{87}{237} \times £100,000$	(36,709)
Chargeable gain	63,291

In this example, had Mr A gone straight to live with friends in July 2001 instead of having six months' occupation, he would have lost not only the extra six months but also the period from July 1997 to June 2002. This period of absence would lose its status of deemed occupation as the property would not have been occupied again by the owner prior to sale.

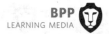

Activity 1: Principal private residence relief

Harry bought his house in London on 1 April 1990 and lived in it until 1 April 1991. From that date until 1 April 1993, he was required by his employers to work overseas.

He returned to the UK on 1 April 1993 to work for his employers in Bristol but lived in rented accommodation there as it was too far to travel daily from London to Bristol to work. He returned to the house on 1 April 1996 for 6 months. From then on, he moved out to go and live with his mother where he remained until he sold his house on 30 September 2016, realising a gain of £100,000.

Required

Complete the following sentence:

The gain on the disposal of his house is £ _____ .

2 Tax planning

For most of the periods of deemed residence a taxpayer has to occupy the property before and after the period of absence. It is vital therefore that the taxpayer returns to the property after a period of absence to ensure they get the exemption. Also, if a taxpayer moves away and plans to sell the house they should try to do it within the eighteen month window to prevent a gain accruing.

Chapter summary

- Any gain arising on the disposal of an individual's principal private residence is exempt from CGT if the individual has occupied/deemed to have occupied the property throughout the period of ownership. A loss on disposal is not allowable.

- If there have been periods of non-occupation, then part of any gain on disposal may be chargeable.

- Certain periods of non-occupation count as periods of deemed occupation.

- The last 18 months of ownership always count as a period of occupation if, at some time, the residence has been the taxpayer's main residence.

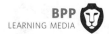

Keywords

- **Deemed occupation:** periods during which an individual is treated as having occupied a residence

- **Principal private residence:** an individual's only or main residence

Activity answers

Activity 1: Principal private residence relief

The gain on the disposal of his house is £ | 69,811 |.

Workings:

PPR – periods of absence	Occ. (mths)	Non-occ (mths)	
1.4.90–31.3.91			
(occupation)	12		
1.4.91–31.3.93			
(working overseas)	24		
1.4.93–31.3.96			
(up to 4 years working in UK)	36		
1.4.96–30.9.96			
(occupation)	6		
1.10.96–31.3.15			
(no deemed occupation as property not reoccupied)		222	
1.4.15–30.9.16			
(Last 18 months)	18		
	96	222	= 318

Capital gain	£
Gain	100,000
Less PPR	
$100,000 \times \dfrac{96}{318}$	(30,189)
Gain	69,811

1   Provided the property has at some time been the owner's principal private residence, the last .... months of ownership is always an exempt period.

Tick ONE box.

	✓
12	
18	
24	
36	

2   **Explain three examples of periods of absence from a property which are deemed periods of occupation for the CGT principal private residence exemption.**

3   Josephine purchased a house on 1 April 1999 for £60,000 and used it as her main residence until 1 August 2002 when she was sent by her employer to manage the Paris office. She worked and lived in Paris until 31 July 2006. Josephine returned to live in the house on 1 August 2006 but moved out to live in a new house (to be treated as her main residence) on 1 May 2008. The property was empty until sold on 30 November 2016 for £180,000.

Using the proforma below, compute the gain on sale.

	£
Proceeds	
Cost	
Gain before PPR exemption	
PPR exemption	
Chargeable gain	

4 Noddy is selling his main residence, which he has owned for 25 years. He lived in the house for the first 14 years of ownership then, for the next 5 years, he was posted abroad by his employer. He never returned to live in the house during the remainder of his period of ownership.

What fraction of his gain will be exempt under the private residence exemption?

Tick ONE box.

	✓
20.5/25	
14/25	
15.5/25	
19/25	

5 Clare bought herself a flat in April 2011 for £80,000. She lived in the flat until December 2015 when she moved to a farmhouse she had bought to be her main residence. The flat was empty until it was sold in March 2017 for £300,000.

Decide whether the following statement is true or false.

Tick ONE box.

The gain arising on the sale is completely exempt.

	✓
True	
False	

Test your learning: answers

Chapter 1 The tax and ethical framework

1

	True ✓	False ✓
All taxpayers are sent a tax return each year by HM Revenue & Customs.		✓

Most taxpayers are employees who have their tax deducted at source under PAYE so they do not need to complete a tax return.

2

	✓
The Chancellor of the Exchequer	
Companies House	
HM Revenue & Customs	✓
Members of Parliament	

3

	✓
Acts of Parliament	✓
HMRC statements of practice	
Statutory instruments	✓
Extra statutory concessions	

4

	✓
When in a social environment	
When discussing client affairs with third parties with the client's proper and specific authority	✓
When reading documents relating to the a client's affairs in public places	
When preparing tax returns	

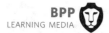

5

	✓
HMRC	
Nearest police station	
National Crime Agency	✓
Tax tribunal	

6 You should tell Cornelius that under the AAT guidelines on client confidentiality, you cannot provide him with any information on another client without the specific authority of that client.

7

	✓
Tax planning	✓
Tax avoidance	
Tax evasion	
Not possible to say until decided by a judge	

8

	✓
Progressive	
Regressive	
Proportional	✓
Equitable	

9

	✓
Not resident or domiciled	
Not resident but domiciled	✓
Resident but not domiciled	
Resident and domiciled	

By leaving the UK he has lost his residence status. He will only lose his domicile status if he takes active steps to show he plans to never return to the UK.

10

	✓
Taxed on all of his income in the UK regardless as to where it is earned	
Taxed in the UK on his UK income and income brought into the UK from overseas	
Taxed in the UK only on his UK income	✓
Not taxed in the UK	

Pierre is not in the UK long enough to be resident. He has never come to the UK before so he cannot be domiciled. He will therefore only be taxed on UK income, for example, the interest earned on his UK bank account.

Chapter 2 National Insurance

1 The class 1 primary National Insurance is £ 4,073

The class 1 secondary National Insurance is £ 4,677

The Class 1A National Insurance is £ 1,104

Workings:

Class 1 Primary
Robert suffers Class 1 primary contributions on his cash earnings.
There is no National Insurance on his reimbursed expenses.

Class 1 – primary
$(42,000 - 8,060) \times 12\% =$ 4,073

Class 1 Secondary
Class 1 – secondary
$(42,000 - 8,112) \times 13.8\% =$ 4,677

Class 1A
8,000 @ 13.8% =   1,104

2

Alec's primary contributions are £ 3,610

Alec's secondary contributions are £ 5,229

Monthly salary 36,000 / 12 = 3,000
March receipt 3,000 + 10,000 = 13,000

Primary contributions

	£
11 months	
£(3,000 – 672) = £2,328 × 12% × 11 (main only)	3,073
1 month (March)	
£(3,583 – 672) = £2,911 × 12% (main)	349
£(13,000 – 3,583) = £9,417 × 2% (additional)	188
Total primary contributions	3,610

Secondary contributions

	£
11 months	
£(3,000 – 676) = £2,324 × 13.8% × 11	3,528
1 month (March)	
£(13,000 – 676) = £12,324 × 13.8%	1,701
Total secondary contributions	5,229

3 Elizabeth's primary contributions are £ | 4,253 |

Elizabeth's secondary contributions are £ | 5,229 |

Elizabeth is a director so her National Insurance is calculated on a cumulative basis. This means that the calculation can be done on an annual basis.

Her annual earnings are £36,000 + £10,000 = £46,000

Primary contributions

	£
£(43,000 – 8,060) = £34,940 × 12% (main)	4,193
£(46,000 – 43,000) = £3,000 × 2% (additional)	60
Total primary contributions	4,253

Secondary contributions

	£
£(46,000 – 8,112) = £37,888 × 13.8%	5,229

4 The Class 1 secondary contributions payable by Ursa Minor Beta Ltd are
£ | 6,492 |

	£
Employee 1: £(25,000 – 8,112) = 16,888 × 13.8%	2,331
Employee 2: £(60,000 – 8,112) = 51,888 × 13.8%	7,161
	9,492
Less employment allowance (maximum)	(3,000)
Secondary contributions 2016/17	6,492

5 If the mileage allowance is 35p a mile the amount subject to class 1 National Insurance is £ | nil |

If the mileage allowance is 50p a mile the amount subject to class 1 National Insurance is £ | 925 |

Workings

If the mileage allowance is 35p

	£
Mileage allowance received (18,500 × 35p)	6,475
Permitted payment (18,500 × 45p)	(8,325)
Excess over limit	0

As the payment is within the permitted amount there is no charge to National Insurance

(b)

	£
Mileage allowance received (18,500 × 50p)	9,250
Less tax free amount (above)	(8,325)
Excess over limit	925

As the payment is above the permitted amount the excess of £925 will be chargeable to class 1 National Insurance, primary and secondary

Chapter 3 Inheritance tax

1

	✓
£150,000	✓
£270,000	
£80,000	
£120,000	

	£
Before the gift: 70% shareholding	350,000
After the gift: 50% shareholding	(200,000)
Transfer of value	150,000

2

	✓
£325,000	
£452,800	
£461,250	✓
£536,250	

	£
Sunita's unused nil rate band £325,000 × 65%	211,250
Joel's nil rate band	325,000
	536,250
Less used against Joel's PET now chargeable	(75,000)
Available nil rate band to set against Joel's death estate	461,250

3

	✓
£28,250	
£31,250	
£29,750	✓
£23,800	

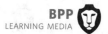

	£
Gift	190,000
Less AE × 2 (15/16 + 14/15 b/f)	(6,000)
	184,000
Less nil rate band available £(£325,000 − 260,000)	(65,000)
	119,000
IHT @ $^{20}/_{80}$	£29,750

4

	✓
£21,000	
Nil	✓
£2,000	
£19,000	

The gift to the granddaughter is covered by the marriage exemption of £2,500 by a remoter ancestor. There was no gratuitous intent on the sale at undervalue of the vase so there is no charge to inheritance tax on this transaction.

5

	✓
£170,000	
£88,000	
£136,000	✓
£132,160	

	£
PET on 10.7.13 PET now chargeable	600,000
Less nil rate band available £(£325,000 − 150,000)	(175,000)
	425,000
IHT @ 40%	170,000
Less taper relief (3 to 4 years) @ 20%	(34,000)
Death tax payable on lifetime transfer	136,000

The chargeable lifetime transfer on 15 September 2009 is cumulated with the later PET since it was made in the 7 years before that transfer

6

	✓
£9,350	
£100	
£9,000	
£350	✓

The gifts to the grandson are exempt as normal expenditure out of income because they are part of the normal expenditure of the donor, made out of income and left the donor with sufficient income to maintain her usual standard of living.

The small gifts exemption only applies to gifts up to £250 per donee per tax year. If gifts total more than £250 the whole amount is chargeable. Since the gifts to the grandnephew totalled £(100 + 250) = £350 in 2016/17, this exemption does not apply.

7

	✓
£123,000	
£27,000	
£66,000	✓
£18,000	

	£
Before the gift: 100% shareholding 1,000 × £150	150,000
After the gift: 70% shareholding 700 × £120	(84,000)
Transfer of value	66,000

8   £24,000

	£
House (net of mortgage) £(200,000 – 60,000)	140,000
Investments and cash	350,000
	490,000
Less funeral expenses	(5,000)
	485,000
Less exempt gift to spouse	(100,000)
Chargeable death estate	385,000
Less available nil rate band (no lifetime transfers)	(325,000)
	60,000
IHT @ 40%	24,000

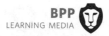

9 $\boxed{£351,000}$

	£
Cash to nephews £200 × 5	1,000
ISA investments	350,000
Chargeable estate	351,000

The small gifts exemption only applies to lifetime transfers. The ISA exemption only applies for income tax and capital gains tax. The residue to the wife is covered by the spouse exemption.

10

Lifetime tax	Death tax	✓
Ruth	Ruth's estate	
Ruth	Trustees	✓
Trustees	Ruths's estate	
Trustees	Trustees	

The tax rate of 20/80 shows that Ruth paid the tax on the lifetime transfer. The recipient always pays the death tax on the lifetime gift.

Chapter 4 Employment income

1. | for services | | of service |

2. | wholly | | exclusively | | necessarily |

3. £ | 5,900 |

Working

	£
Amount received: 8,000 × 35p	2,800
Less statutory limit: 8,000 × 45p	(3,600)
Deductible amount	(800)

4. £ | 5,900 |

being the higher of the annual value and rent actually paid by the employer.

5.

	✓
True	
False	✓

There is a taxable fuel benefit unless the employer is fully reimbursed for private fuel.

6.

	✓
£325	
£400	
£175	
£250	✓

Working

The benefit is the higher of:

		£	£
(a)	Current MV	325	
(b)	Original MV	500	
	Less already assessed (in 2016/17)		
	£500 × 20%	(100)	
		400	
			400
	Less amount paid		(150)
	Taxable benefit		250

7

	✓
True	
False	✓

Only if total loans do not exceed £10,000 at any time in the tax year are they ignored.

8 £ | 6,480 |

Working

CO_2 emissions = 150 g/km (rounded down)
Above baseline: 150 – 95 = 55 g/km
Divide by 5 = 55/5 = 11
Percentage = 16% + 11% = 27%
Benefit 27% × £24,000 = £6,480

9 £ | 28,260 |

	£
Car benefit (W)	21,600
Fuel benefit (£22,200 × 30%)	6,660
Telephone benefit (exempt – one mobile phone)	Nil
Total benefit	28,260

Working

Amount of emissions above baseline: 165 – 95 = 70 g/km
Divide 70 by 5 = 14
Percentage = 16% + 14% = 30%
£72,000 × 30% = £21,600

10

Item	Taxable	Exempt
Write off loan of £8,000 (only loan provided)	✓	☐
Payments by employer of £500 per month into registered pension scheme	☐	✓
Provision of one mobile phone	☐	✓
Provision of a company car for both business and private use	✓	☐
Removal costs of £5,000 paid to an employee relocating to another branch	☐	✓
Accommodation provided to enable the employee to spend longer time in the office	✓	☐

Chapter 5 Property income

1 £ [1,200]

Rent accrued 1 December 2016 to 5 April 2017 = 4/12 × £3,600

2 £ [5,000]

Working

Insurance premiums accrued in 2016/17:

	£
6/12 × £4,800 (6 April 2016 to 30 September 2016)	2,400
6/12 × £5,200 (1 October 2016 to 5 April 2017)	2,600
	5,000

3 £ [1,667]

Working

	£
Rental income (£4,000 × 8/12)	2,667
Less expenses	(1,000)
Taxable rental income	1,667

Rent of £5,000, paid on 4 April 2017 accrues in 2017/18 and is therefore taxed in that year.

4 To minimise their tax liability the property should be [held in Ben's name]

Polly is paying tax at 45%, Ben is paying tax at 20% so if the asset is held by Polly she will pay tax of £12,000 x 45% = £5,400 whereas if the asset is held by Ben he will pay tax of £12,000 x 20% = £2,400 saving them together £3,000.

5

	✓
Carried back one year and offset against property income only	
Offset against net income in the current year	
Carried forward for one year only and offset against property income	
Carried forward indefinitely and offset against property income only	✓

Chapter 6 Taxable income

1

	Non-savings income	Savings income	Dividend income
Employment income	✓	☐	☐
Dividends	☐	☐	✓
Property income	✓	☐	☐
Bank interest	☐	✓	☐
Pension income	✓	☐	☐
Interest on government stock	☐	✓	☐

2

	Amount received £	Amount in tax return £
Building society interest	240	240
Interest on an individual savings account	40	0
Dividends	160	160
Interest from government gilts	350	350

3

	Non-savings income £	Dividend income £	Total £
Employment income	30,000		30,000
Dividends		300	300
Net income	30,000	300	30,300
Less personal allowance	(11,000)		(11,000)
Taxable income	19,000	300	19,300

Premium bond winnings are exempt from income tax.

4

	Non-savings income £	Savings income £	Total £
Property income	3,000		3,000
Building society interest		9,000	9,000
Net income	3,000	9,000	12,000
Less personal allowance	(3,000)	(8,000)	(11,000)
Taxable income	Nil	1,000	1,000

The personal allowance is deducted first from non-savings income and then from savings income.

5

	Non-savings income £	Savings income £	Dividend income £	Total £
Employment income	112,200			112,200
Building society interest		5,000		5,000
Dividends			4,000	4,000
Net income	112,200	5,000	4,000	121,200
Less personal allowance (W)	(400)			(400)
Taxable income	111,800	5,000	4,000	120,800

Working

	£
Net income	121,200
Less income limit	(100,000)
Excess	21,200
Personal allowance	11,000
Less half excess	(10,600)
Adjusted personal allowance	400

The prize is exempt from income tax.

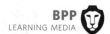

Chapter 7 Calculation of income tax

1

	✓
0%, 20%, 40% and 45%	
40% and 45%	
20% only	
20%, 40% and 45%	✓

2   £ 1,320

Working

	Non-savings income £	Savings income £	Dividend income £	Total £
Net income	16,600	2,000	3,000	21,600
Less personal allowance	(11,000)	–	–	(11,000)
Taxable income	5,600	2,000	3,000	10,600

	£
Tax on non-savings income	
5,600 × 20%	1,120
Tax on savings income	
1,000 × 0%	0
1,000 × 20%	200
Tax on dividend income	
3,000 × 0%	0
Tax liability	1,320

Albert is a basic rate taxpayer so has a personal savings allowance of £1,000. The dividend allowance is always £5,000.

3   £ 3,075

Working

	Non-savings income £	Savings income £	Dividend income £	Total £
Employment income	5,000			5,000
Interest		18,000		18,000
Dividends			22,000	22,000
Net income	5,000	18,000	22,000	45,000
Less personal allowance	(5,000)	(6,000)		(11,000)
Taxable income	Nil	12,000	22,000	34,000

Tax on savings income	£
5,000 × 0%	0
500 × 0%	0
6,500 × 20%	1,300
12,000	

	£
Tax on dividend income	
5,000 × 0%	0
15,000 × 7.5%	1,125
32,000	
2,000 × 32.5%	650
34,000	
Income tax liability	3,075

Net income is > £43,000 < £151,000 so personal savings allowance of £500 available. Dividend allowance of £5,000 always available.

4 £ 67,625

Working

	Non-savings income £	Savings income £	Dividend income £	Total £
Employment income	140,000			140,000
Interest		20,000		20,000
Dividends			30,000	30,000
Net income	140,000	20,000	30,000	190,000
Less personal allowance	(Nil)			(Nil)
Taxable income	140,000	20,000	30,000	190,000

The personal allowance and personal savings allowance are nil because the net income is so high.

	£
Tax on non-savings income	
32,000 × 20%	6,400
108,000 × 40%	43,200
140,000	
Tax on savings income	
10,000 × 40%	4,000
150,000	
10,000 × 45%	4,500
160,000	

			£
Tax on dividend income			
5,000 × 0%			0
25,000 × 38.1%			9,525
190,000			
Income tax liability			67,625

5 Basic rate tax relief is obtained by paying Gift Aid donations net of 20% tax. Further tax relief is given to higher and additional rate taxpayers by extending the basic and higher rate bands by the gross amount of the Gift Aid donation.

6

	Non-savings income	Savings income	Dividend income	Total
	£	£	£	£
Pension income	17,000			17,000
Property income	3,500			3,500
Interest (received gross)		380		380
Dividends			700	700
Net income	20,500	380	700	21,580
Less personal allowance	(11,000)			(11,000)
Taxable income	9,500	380	700	10,580

Premium bond prizes are exempt from income tax. She is a basic rate taxpayer so receives the full personal savings allowance of £1,000. The £5,000 dividend allowance is also available.

	£
Tax on non-savings income	
£9,500 × 20%	1,900
Tax on savings income	
£380 × 0%	0
Tax on dividend income	
£700 × 0%	0
	1,900
Less tax deducted from pension income (given)	(2,010)
Income tax repayable	(110)

7

	Non-savings income £	Savings income £	Dividend income £	Total £
Business profits	36,600			36,600
Building society interest		2,000		2,000
Dividends			8,000	8,000
Net income	36,600	2,000	8,000	46,600
Less personal allowance	(11,000)			(11,000)
Taxable income	25,600	2,000	8,000	35,600

	£
Tax on non-savings income	
£25,600 × 20%	5,120
Tax on savings income	
£500 × 0%	0
£1,500 × 20%	300
Tax on dividend income	
£5,000 × 0%	0
£1,400 × 7.5%	105
£34,000	
£1,600 × 32.5% (£8,000 – £5,000 – £1,400)	520
Income tax liability/payable	6,045

Note. Gross Gift Aid payment = £1,600 × 100/80 = £2,000. Basic rate extends to £34,000.

Adjusted net income = £46,600 – £2,000 = £44,600 > £43,000 so £500 personal savings allowance available

8

	✓
£32,000	
£47,000	
£50,750	✓
£57,000	

Working

£15,000 × 100/80 = £18,750 + £32,000

Chapter 8 Chargeable gains

1

	Chargeable ✓	Exempt ✓
A gift of an antique necklace	✓	
The sale of a building	✓	
Sale of a racehorse		✓

2

	£
Proceeds of sale	200,000
Less cost	(80,000)
Less enhancement expenditure	(10,000)
Chargeable gain	110,000

3   £ | 144,600 |

£ | 0 |

	£
Gains	171,000
Less current year losses	(5,300)
	165,700
Less losses b/f	(10,000)
	155,700
Less annual exempt amount	(11,100)
Taxable gains	144,600

4   £ | 2,560 |

	£
Chargeable gains	23,900
Less annual exempt amount	(11,100)
Taxable gains	12,800
CGT on £12,800 @ 20%	2,560

5 | 31/01/2018 |

6

	✓
£16,663	✓
£17,500	
£19,663	
£18,337	

	£
Proceeds	38,000
Less costs of disposal	(3,000)
	35,000
Less £41,500 × $\frac{38,000}{38,000+48,000}$	(18,337)
Chargeable gain	16,663

7

(a)

£	Nil

There is no gain as the chattel cost and gross proceeds are both less than £6,000.

(b)

£	4,033

	£
Gross proceeds	8,420
Less selling expenses	(220)
Net proceeds	8,200
Less cost	(3,500)
	4,700

Gain cannot exceed 5/3 (8,420 – 6,000) = £4,033

Therefore, gain is £4,033

8

	✓
True	
False	✓

A loss on a disposal to a connected person can be set only against gains arising on disposals to the same connected person.

9

	✓
True	✓
False	

10

	Actual proceeds used	Deemed proceeds (market value) used	No gain or loss basis
Paul sells an asset to his civil partner Joe for £3,600.			✓
Grandmother gives an asset to her grandchild worth £1,000.		✓	
Sarah sells an asset worth £20,000 to her best friend Cathy for £12,000. Sarah knows the asset is worth £20,000.		✓	

Chapter 9 Share disposals

1

	✓
£15,750	
£11,500	
£17,000	
£14,250	✓

	No of shares	Cost
		£
August 1994 acquisition	10,000	5,000
April 2009 acquisition	10,000	16,000
	20,000	21,000
November 2016 disposal	(15,000)	(15,750)
(£21,000 × 15,000/20,000 = £15,750)		
c/f	5,000	5,250

	£
Proceeds of sale	30,000
Less allowable cost	(15,750)
Chargeable gain	14,250

2

	✓
True	
False	✓

In a rights issue, shares are paid for and this amount is added to the original cost. In a bonus issue, shares are not paid for and so there is no adjustment to the original cost.

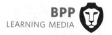

3 £ [3,750]

	No of shares	Cost £
May 2003 acquisition	2,000	12,000
December 2004 1 for 2 rights issue @ £7.50	1,000	7,500
(1/2 × 2,000 = 1,000 shares × £7.50 = £7,500)		
	3,000	19,500
March 2017 disposal	(2,500)	(16,250)
(£19,500 × 2,500/3,000)		
c/f	500	3,250

	£
Proceeds of sale	20,000
Less allowable costs	(16,250)
Chargeable gain	3,750

4 £ [7,000]

	No of shares	Cost £
June 2011 acquisition	6,000	15,000
August 2012 1 for 3 bonus issue		
(1/3 × 6,000 = 2,000 shares)	2,000	nil
	8,000	15,000
December 2016 disposal (ie all the shares)	(8,000)	(15,000)
c/f	nil	nil

	£
Proceeds of sale	22,000
Less allowable costs	(15,000)
Chargeable gain	7,000

5   The matching rules for shares disposed of are:

(a)   Shares acquired on the same day
(b)   Shares acquired in the next 30 days
(c)   Shares from the share pool

Chapter 10 Principal private residence

1

	✓
12	
18	✓
24	
36	

2

The last 18 months of ownership is deemed occupation if, at some time, the residence has been the taxpayer's main residence.

Providing the taxpayer actually occupies the property both at some point before and at some point after the period of absence, the following periods are deemed occupation for the purpose of PPR exemption:

(a) Periods of up to three years for any reason. Where a period of absence exceeds three years, three years out of the longer period are deemed to be a period of occupation.

(b) Periods during which the owner was required by their employment to live abroad.

(c) Period of up to four years where the owner was:

(i) Self-employed and forced to work away from home (UK and abroad)

(ii) Employed and required to work elsewhere in the UK (overseas employment is covered by (b) above)

3

	£
Proceeds	180,000
Cost	(60,000)
Gain before PPR exemption	120,000
PPR exemption 127/212 × £120,000	(71,887)
Chargeable gain	48,113

Working

Total period of ownership: 1 April 1999 to 30 November 2016 = 17 years and 8 months (212 months)

	Exempt months	Chargeable months
1 April 1999 to 31 July 2002 (actual occupation)	40	
1 August 2002 to 31 July 2006 (employed abroad)	48	
1 August 2006 to 30 April 2008 (actual occupation)	21	
1 May 2008 to 31 May 2015		85
1 June 2015 to 30 November 2016 (last 18 months)	18	—
	127	85

Exempt 127/212 × £120,000 = £71,887

4

	✓
20.5/25	
14/25	
15.5/25	✓
19/25	

The five years posted abroad will not be deemed occupation as he never returned to live in the property. Therefore, only the actual 14 years of occupation and the last 18 months of ownership will be exempt.

5

	✓
True	✓
False	

Clare was in actual occupation from April 2011 to December 2015.

The last 18 months of ownership are exempt because Clare had previously lived in the flat as her only or main residence. Therefore, this covers her period of absence from December 2015 to March 2017.

Tax tables 2016/2017

Tax rates and bands

Rates	Bands	Normal rates (%)	Dividend rates (%)
Basic rate	£1 – £32,000	20	7.5
Higher rate	£32,001 – £150,000	40	32.5
Additional rate	£150,001 and over	45	38.1

		£
Personal allowance		11,000
Savings allowances:	Basic rate tax payer	1,000
	Higher rate tax payer	500
Dividend allowance		5,000
Income limit for personal allowances		100,000

Individual savings accounts

	£
Annual limit	15,240

Car benefit percentage

		%
Emissions for petrol engines:	0g/kilometre to 50g/km	7
	51g/km to 75g/km	11
	76g/km to 94g/km	15
	95g/km or more	16 + 1% for every extra 5g/km above 95g/km
Diesel engines		Additional 3%
Electric vehicles		7

Car fuel benefit

Car fuel benefit	£
Base figure	22,200

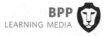

Approved mileage allowance payments

Mileage	Payment
First 10,000 miles	45p per mile
Over 10,000 miles	25p per mile
Additional passengers (per passenger)	5p per mile
Motorcycles	24p per mile
Bicycles	20p per mile

Van scale charge

	£
Basic charge	3,170
Private fuel charge	598
	%
Benefit charge for zero emissions vans	20

Other benefits in kind

Staff party or event		£150 per head
Incidental overnight expenses:	Within the UK	£5 per night
	Overseas	£10 per night
Removal or relocation expenses		£8,000
Non-cash gifts from someone other than the employer		£250 per tax year
Staff suggestion scheme		Up to £5,000
Non-cash long service award		£50 per year of service
Tax-free pay whilst attending a full time course		£15,480 per academic year
Health screening		1 per year
Mobiles telephones		1 per employee

Childcare provision:	Basic rate taxpayer	£55 per week
	Higher rate taxpayer	£28 per week
	Additional rate taxpayer	£25 per week
Low-rate or interest free loans		Up to £10,000
Subsidised meals		£Nil
Provision of parking spaces		£Nil
Provision of workplace childcare		£Nil
Provision of workplace sports facilities		£Nil
Provision of eye tests and spectacles for VDU use		£Nil
Job-related accommodation		£Nil
Expensive accommodation limit		£75,000
Loan of assets annual charge		20%

HMRC official rate

HMRC official rate	3%

National Insurance contributions

		%
Class 1 Employee:	£1 to £8,060	0
	£8,061 to £43,000	12
	£43,001 and above	2
Class 1 Employer:	£1 to 8,112	0
	£8,113 and above	13.8
Class 1A		13.8
		£
Employment allowance		3,000

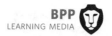

Capital gains tax and tax rates

Capital gains tax	£
Annul exempt amount	11,100
Tax rates	**%**
Basic rate	10
High rate	20

Inheritance tax – tax rates

		%
£1 to £325,000		0
Excess:	Death rate	40
	Lifetime rate	20

Inheritance tax – taper relief

	% reduction
3 years or less	0
Over 3 years but less than 4 years	20
Over 4 years but less than 5 years	40
Over 5 years but less than 6 years	60
Over 6 years but less than 7 years	80

Inheritance tax – exemptions

		£
Small gifts		250 per transferee per tax year
Marriage or civil partnership:	From a parent	5,000
	From a grandparent	2,500
	From one party to the other	2,500
	From others	1,000
Annual exemption		3,000

Reference material

Interpretation and abbreviations

Context

Tax advisers operate in a complex business and financial environment. The increasing public focus on the role of taxation in wider society means a greater interest in the actions of tax advisers and their clients.

This guidance, written by the professional bodies for their members working in tax, sets out the hallmarks of a good tax adviser, and in particular the fundamental principles of behaviour that members are expected to follow.

Interpretation

1.1 In this guidance:

- 'Client' includes, where the context requires, 'former client'.

- 'Member' (and 'members') includes 'firm' or 'practice' and the staff thereof.

- For simplicity, 'she' and 'her' are used throughout but should be taken to include 'he' and 'his'.

- Words in the singular include the plural and words in the plural include the singular.

Abbreviations

1.2 The following abbreviations have been used:

CCAB	Consultative Committee of Accountancy Bodies
DOTAS	Disclosure of Tax Avoidance Schemes
GAAP	Generally Accepted Accounting Principles
GAAR	General Anti-Abuse Rule in Finance Act 2013
HMRC	Her Majesty's Revenue and Customs
MLRO	Money Laundering Reporting Officer
NCA	National Crime Agency (previously the Serious Organised Crime Agency, SOCA)
POTAS	Promoters of Tax Avoidance Schemes
SRN	Scheme Reference Number

Fundamental principles

Overview of the fundamental principles

2.1 Ethical behaviour in the tax profession is critical. The work carried out by a member needs to be trusted by society at large as well as by clients and other stakeholders. What a member does reflects not just on themselves but on the profession as a whole.

2.2 A member must comply with the following fundamental principles:

Integrity

To be straightforward and honest in all professional and business relationships.

Objectivity

To not allow bias, conflict of interest or undue influence of others to override professional or business judgements.

Professional competence and due care

To maintain professional knowledge and skill at the level required to ensure that a client or employer receives competent professional service based on current developments in practice, legislation and techniques and act diligently and in accordance with applicable technical and professional standards.

Confidentiality

To respect the confidentiality of information acquired as a result of professional and business relationships and, therefore, not disclose any such information to third parties without proper and specific authority, unless there is a legal or professional right or duty to disclose, nor use the information for the personal advantage of the member or third parties.

Professional behaviour

To comply with relevant laws and regulations and avoid any action that discredits the profession.

Each of these fundamental principles is discussed in more detail in the context of taxation services.

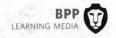

Tax return

Definition of tax return (return)

3.1 For the purposes of this Chapter, the term 'return' includes any document or online submission of data that is prepared on behalf of the client for the purposes of disclosing to any taxing authority details that are to be used in the calculation of tax due by a client or a refund of tax due to the client or for other official purposes and, for example, includes:

- Self-assessment returns for income or corporation tax;

- VAT and Customs returns;

- PAYE returns;

- Inheritance tax returns;

- Returns or claims in respect of any other tax or duties where paid to the UK Government or any authority, such as a devolved government.

3.2 A letter giving details in respect of a return or as an amendment to a return including, for example, any voluntary disclosure on an error should be dealt with as if it was a return.

Taxpayer's responsibility

3.3 The taxpayer has primary responsibility to submit correct and complete returns to the best of her knowledge and belief. The return may include reasonable estimates where necessary. It follows that the final decision as to whether to disclose any issue is that of the client.

Member's responsibility

3.4 A member who prepares a return on behalf of a client is responsible to the client for the accuracy of the return based on the information provided.

3.5 In dealing with HMRC in relation to a client's tax affairs a member must bear in mind her duty of confidentiality to the client and that she is acting as the agent of her client. She has a duty to act in the best interests of her client.

3.6 A member must act in good faith in dealings with HMRC in accordance with the fundamental principle of integrity. In particular the member must take reasonable care and exercise appropriate professional scepticism when making statements or asserting facts on behalf of a client. Where acting as a tax agent, a member is not required to audit the figures in the books and records provided or verify information provided by a client or by a third party. A member should take care not to be associated with the presentation of facts she knows or believes to be incorrect or misleading nor to assert tax positions in a tax return which she considers have no sustainable basis.

3.7 When a member is communicating with HMRC, she should consider whether she needs to make it clear to what extent she is relying on information which has been supplied by the client or a third party.

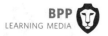

Materiality

3.8 Whether an amount is to be regarded as material depends upon the facts and circumstances of each case.

3.9 The profits of a trade, profession, vocation or properly business must be computed in accordance with GAAP subject to any adjustment required or authorised by law in computing profits for those purposes. This permits a trade, profession, vocation or property business to disregard non-material adjustments in computing its accounting profits. However, it should be noted that for certain small businesses an election may be made to use the cash basis instead.

3.10 The application of GAAP, and therefore materiality, does not extend beyond the accounting profits. Thus the accounting concept of materiality cannot be applied when completing tax returns (direct and indirect), for example when:

- Computing adjustments required to accounting figures so as to arrive at taxable profits;
- Allocating income, expenses and outgoings across the relevant boxes on a self-assessment tax return;
- Collating the aggregate figures from all shareholdings and bank accounts for disclosure on tax returns.

Disclosure

3.11 If a client is unwilling to include in a tax return the minimum information required by law, the member should follow the guidance in Chapter 5 Irregularities. 3.12–3.18 give guidance on some of the more common areas of uncertainty over disclosure.

3.12 In general, it is likely to be in a client's own interests to ensure that factors relevant to her tax liability are adequately disclosed to HMRC because:

- Her relationship with HMRC is more likely to be on a satisfactory footing if she can demonstrate good faith in her dealings with them; and
- She will reduce the risk of a discovery or further assessment and may reduce exposure to interest and penalties.

3.13 It may be advisable to consider fuller disclosure than is strictly necessary. The factors involved in making this decision include:

- The terms of the applicable law;
- The view taken by the member;
- The extent of any doubt that exists;
- The manner in which disclosure is to be made; and
- The size and gravity of the item in question.

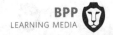

3.14 When advocating fuller disclosure than is strictly necessary a member should ensure that her client is adequately aware of the issues involved and their potential implications. Fuller disclosure should not be made unless the client consents to the level of disclosure.

3.15 Cases will arise where there is doubt as to the correct treatment of an item of income or expenditure, or the computation of a gain or allowance. In such cases a member ought to consider carefully what disclosure, if any, might be necessary. For example, additional disclosure should be considered where:

- A return relies on a valuation;

- There is inherent doubt as to the correct treatment of an item, for example, expenditure on repairs which might be regarded as capital in whole or part, or the VAT liability of a particular transaction; or

- HMRC has published its interpretation or has indicated its practice on a point, but the client proposes to adopt a different view, whether or not supported by Counsel's opinion. The member should refer to the guidance on the Veltema case and 3.19.

3.16 A member who is uncertain whether her client should disclose a particular item or of its treatment should consider taking further advice before reaching a decision. She should use her best endeavours to ensure that the client understands the issues, implications and the proposed course of action. Such a decision may have to be justified at a later date, so the member's files should contain sufficient evidence to support the position taken, including contemporaneous notes of discussions with the client and/or with other advisers, copies of any second opinion obtained and the client's final decision. A failure to take reasonable care may result in HMRC imposing a penalty if an error is identified after an enquiry.

3.17 The 2012 case of *Charlton* clarified the law on discovery in relation to tax schemes disclosed to HMRC under DOTAS. The Upper Tribunal made clear that where the taxpayer has:

(i) Disclosed details of a significant allowable loss claim;

(ii) Declared relatively modest income/gains; and/or

(iii) Included the SRN issued by HMRC on the appropriate self-assessment tax return,

an HMRC officer of reasonable knowledge and skill would be expected to infer that the taxpayer had entered into a tax avoidance scheme (and that fuller details of such scheme would be contained in the relevant AAG1 Form). As a result, HMRC would be precluded, in most cases, from raising a discovery assessment in a situation where the client implemented the disclosed scheme and HMRC failed to open an enquiry within the required time.

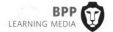

3.18 It is essential where a member is involved in the preparation of a self-assessment tax return which includes a scheme disclosed under DOTAS that the member takes care to ensure:

- That the tax return provides sufficient details of any transactions entered into (in case the AAG1 Form is incomplete);

- That the SRN is recorded properly in the appropriate box included for this purpose on a self-assessment tax return; and

- The SRN is shown for the self-assessment return for each year in which the scheme is expected to give the client a tax advantage.

Supporting documents

3.19 For the most part, HMRC does not consider that it is necessary for a taxpayer to provide supporting documentation in order to satisfy the taxpayer's overriding need to make a correct return. HMRC's view is that, where it is necessary for that purpose, explanatory information should be entered in the 'white space' provided on the return. However, HMRC does recognise that the taxpayer may wish to supply further details of a particular computation or transaction in order to minimise the risk of a discovery assessment being raised at a later time.

3.20 Further HMRC guidance says that sending attachments with a tax return is intended for those cases where the taxpayer 'feels it is crucial to provide additional information to support the return but for some reason cannot utilise the white space'.

Approval of tax returns

3.21 It is essential that the member advises the client to review her tax return before it is submitted.

3.22 The member should draw the client's attention to the responsibility which the client is taking in approving the return as correct and complete. Attention should be drawn to any judgemental areas or positions reflected in the return to ensure that the client is aware of these and their implications before she approves the return.

3.23 A member should obtain evidence of the client's approval of the return in electronic or non-electronic form.

Tax advice

Introduction

4.1 Giving tax advice covers a variety of activities. It can involve advising a client on a choice afforded to her by legislation, for example, whether to establish a business as a sole trader, partnership or company. It could be advising on the tax implications of buying or selling an asset or business, or advising on succession planning.

4.2 For the most part clients are seeking advice on how to structure their affairs, either personal or commercial, in a way that is tax efficient and ensures that they comply with their legal and regulatory requirements. Transactions based on advice which are centred around non-tax objectives are less likely to attract scrutiny or criticism from stakeholders and are much more likely to withstand challenge by HMRC.

4.3 Some tax strategies have been the subject of heated public debate, raising ethical challenges. Involvement in certain arrangements could subject the client and the member to significantly greater compliance requirements, scrutiny or investigation as well as criticism from the media, government and other stakeholders and difficulties in obtaining professional indemnity insurance cover.

4.4 The definition of 'avoidance' is an evolving area that can depend on the tax legislation, the intention of Parliament, interpretations in case law and the varying perceptions of different stakeholders and is discussed further below.

4.5 A member should consider the contents of this Chapter carefully when giving tax advice and the potential negative impact of her actions on the public perception of the integrity of the tax profession more generally.

4.6 Clearly a member must never be knowingly involved in tax evasion, although, of course, it is appropriate to act for a client who is rectifying their affairs.

Tax planning versus tax avoidance?

4.7 Despite attempts by courts over the years to elucidate tax 'avoidance' and to distinguish this from acceptable tax planning or mitigation, there is no widely accepted definition.

4.8 Publicly, the term 'avoidance' is used in the context of a wide range of activities, be it multinational structuring or entering contrived tax-motivated schemes. The application of one word to a range of activities and behaviours oversimplifies the concept and has led to confusion.

4.9 In a 2012 paper on tax avoidance, the Oxford University Centre for Business Taxation states that transactions generally do not fall into clear categories of tax avoidance, mitigation or planning. Similarly, it is often not clear whether something is acceptable or unacceptable. Instead the paper concludes that there is:

'a continuum from transactions that would not be effective to save tax under the law as it stands at present to tax planning that would be accepted by revenue authorities and courts without question.'

Member's responsibility in giving tax planning advice

4.10 A member is required to act with professional competence and due care within the scope of her engagement letter.

4.11 A member should understand her client's expectations around tax advice or tax planning, and ensure that engagement letters reflect the member's role and responsibilities, including limitations in or amendments to that role. The importance of this has been highlighted by the Mehjoo case.

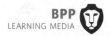

4.12 A member does not have to advise on or recommend tax planning which she does not consider to be appropriate or otherwise does not align with her own business principles and ethics. However, in this situation the member may need to ensure that the advice she does not wish to give is outside the scope of her engagement. If the member may owe a legal duty of care to the client to advise in this area, the member should ensure that she complies with this by, for example, advising the client that there are opportunities that the client could undertake, even though the member is unwilling to assist, and recommending that the client seeks alternative advice. Any such discussions should be well documented by the member.

4.13 Ultimately it is the client's decision as to what planning is appropriate having received advice and taking into account their own broader commercial objectives and ethical stance. However, the member should ensure that the client is made aware of the risks and rewards of any planning, including that there may be adverse reputational consequences. It is advisable to ensure that the basis for recommended tax planning is clearly identified in documentation.

4.14 Occasionally a client may advise a member that she intends to proceed with a tax planning arrangement without taking full advice from her on the relevant issues or despite the advice the member has given. In such cases the member should warn the client of the potential risks of proceeding without full advice and ensure that the restriction in the scope of the member's advice is recorded in writing.

4.15 Where a client wishes to pursue a claim for a tax advantage which the member feels has no sustainable basis the member should refer to Chapter 5 Irregularities for further guidance.

4.16 If Counsel's opinion is sought on the planning the member should consider including the question as to whether, in Counsel's view, the GAAR could apply to the transaction.

4.17 It should be noted that any legal opinion provided, for example by Counsel, will be based on the assumptions stated in the instructions for the opinion and on execution of the arrangement exactly as stated. HMRC and the courts will not be constrained by these assumptions.

The different roles of a Tax Adviser

4.18 A member may be involved in tax planning arrangements in the following ways:

- Advising on a planning arrangement.
- Introducing another adviser's planning arrangement.
- Providing a second opinion on a third party's planning arrangement.
- Compliance services in relation to a return which includes a planning arrangement.

A member should always make a record of any advice given.

Irregularities

Introduction

5.1 For the purposes of this Chapter, the term 'irregularity' is intended to include all errors whether the error is made by the client, the member, HMRC or any other party involved in a client's tax affairs.

5.2 In the course of a member's relationship with the client, the member may become aware of possible irregularities in the client's tax affairs. Unless already aware of the possible irregularities in question, the client should be informed as soon as the member has knowledge of them.

5.3 Where the irregularity has resulted in the client paying too much tax the member should advise the client about making a repayment claim and have regard to any relevant time limits. With the exception of this paragraph, the rest of this Chapter deals solely with situations where sums may be due to HMRC.

5.4 On occasion, it may be apparent that an error made by HMRC has meant that the client has not paid tax actually due or she has been incorrectly repaid tax. Correcting such mistakes may cause expense to a member and thereby to her clients. A member should bear in mind that, in some circumstances, clients or agents may be able to claim for additional professional costs incurred and compensation from HMRC.

5.5 A member must act correctly from the outset. A member should keep sufficient appropriate records of discussions and advice and when dealing with irregularities the member should:

- Give the client appropriate advice;

- If necessary, so long as she continues to act for the client, seek to persuade the client to behave correctly;

- Take care not to appear to be assisting a client to plan or commit any criminal offence or to conceal any offence which has been committed; and

- In appropriate situations, or where in doubt, discuss the client's situation with a colleague or an independent third party.

5.6 Once aware of a possible irregularity, a member must bear in mind the legislation on money laundering and the obligations and duties which this places upon her.

5.7 A member should also consider whether the irregularity could give rise to a circumstance requiring notification to her professional indemnity insurers.

5.8 In any situation where a member has concerns about her own position, she should take specialist legal advice. This might arise, for example, where a client appears to have used the member to assist in the commission of a

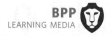

criminal offence in such a way that doubt could arise as to whether the member had acted honestly and in good faith.

5.9 The irregularity steps flowchart (5.10) summarises the recommended steps a member should take where a possible irregularity arises.

5.10 **Steps to take of there is a possible irregularity**

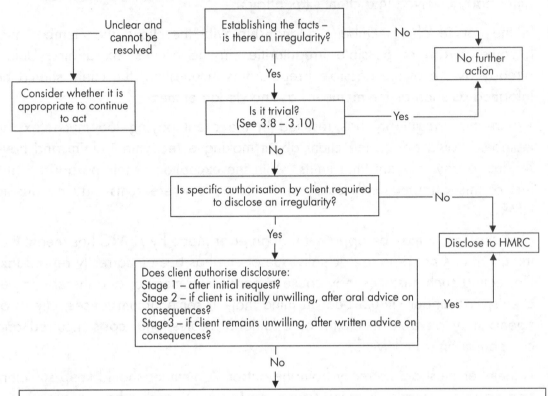

Access to data by HMRC

Introduction

6.1 For the purposes of this Chapter the term 'data' includes documents in whatever form (including electronic) and other information. While this guidance relates to HMRC requests, other government bodies or organisations may also approach the member for data. The same principles apply.

6.2 A distinction must be drawn between a request for data made informally and those requests for data which are made in exercise of a power to require the provision of the data requested ('statutory requests').

6.3   Similarly, requests addressed to a client and those addressed to a member require different handling.

6.4   Where a member no longer acts for a client, the member remains subject to the duty of confidentiality.

6.5   A member should comply with reasonable statutory requests and should not seek to frustrate legitimate requests for information. Adopting a constructive approach may help to resolve issues promptly and minimise costs to all parties.

6.6   Whilst a member should be aware of HMRC's powers in relation to the access, inspection and removal of data, given the complexity of the law relating to information powers, it may be appropriate to take specialist advice.

6.7   Revenue Scotland will have separate powers under the Revenue Scotland and Tax Powers Act 2014.

Informal request addressed to the member

6.8   Disclosure in response to informal request not made under any statutory power to demand data can only be made with the client's permission.

6.9   Sometimes the client will have authorised routine disclosure of relevant data, for example, through the engagement latter. However, if there is any doubt about whether the client has authorised disclosure or about the accuracy of details, the members should ask the client to approve what is to be disclosed.

6.10 Where an oral enquiry is made by HMRC, a member should consider asking for it to be put in writing so that a response may be agreed with the client.

6.11 Although there is no obligation to comply with an informal request in whole or in part, a member should advise the client whether it is in the client's best interests to disclose such data.

6.12 Informal requests may be forerunners to statutory requests compelling the disclosure of data. Consequently, it may be sensible to comply with such requests or to seek to persuade HMRC that a more limited request is appropriate. The member should advise the client as to reasonableness of the informal request and likely consequences of not providing the data, so that the client can decide on her preferred course of action.

Informal requests addressed to the client

6.13 From time to time HMRC chooses to communicate directly with clients rather than with the appointed agent.

6.14 HMRC recognises the significant value which tax agents bring to both their clients and to the operation of the tax system. However, HMRC has also made it clear that on occasions it may deal with the taxpayers as well as, or instead of, the agent.

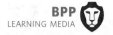

6.15 Examples of where HMRC may contact a member's client directly include:

- Where HMRC is using 'nudge' techniques to encourage taxpayers or claimants to re-check their financial records or to change behaviour.

- Where HMRC has become aware of particular assets, such as offshore investments, and the tax payer is encouraged to consider whether a further tax disclosure is required.

- Where the taxpayers has engaged in what HMRC considers to be a tax avoidance scheme, as HMRC considers that this will better ensure that the client fully understands HMRC's view.

6.16 HMRC has given reassurances that it is working to ensure that initial contact on compliance checks will normally be via the agent and only of the agent does not reply within an appropriate timescale will the contact be direct to the client.

6.17 When the member assists a client in dealing with such requests from HMRC, the member should apply the principles in 6.8 – 6.12.

Statutory requests addressed to the client

6.18 In advising the client a member should consider whether the notice is valid, how to comply the request and the consequences of non-compliance. Specialist advice may be needed, for example on such issues as whether the notice has been issued in accordance with the relevant tax legislation, whether the data requested is validly included in the notice, legal professional privilege and human rights.

6.19 Even if the notice is not valid, in many cases the client may conclude that the practical answer is to comply. If the notice is legally effective the client is legally obliged to comply with the request.

6.20 The member should also advise the client about any relevant right of appeal against the statutory request if appropriate and of the consequences of a failure to comply.

Statutory requests addressed to the member

6.21 The same principles apply to statutory request to the member as statutory requests to clients.

6.22 If a statutory request is valid it override the member's duty of confidentiality to her client.

6.23 In cases where the member is not legally precluded by the terms of the notice from communicating with the client, the members should advise the client of the notice and keep the client informed of progress and developments.

6.24 The member remains under a duty to preserve the confidentiality of her client so care must be taken to ensure that in complying with any notice the member does not provide information or data outside the scope of the notice.

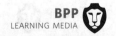

6.25 If a member is faced with a situation is which HMRC is seeking to enforce disclosure by the removal of data, the member should consider seeking immediate advice from a specialist adviser or other practitioner with relevant specialist knowledge, before permitting such removal, to ensure that this is the legally correct course of action.

6.26 Where a Schedule 36 notice is in point a member should note that it does not allow HMRC to inspect business premises occupied by a member in her capacity as an adviser. Specialist advice should be sought in any situation where HMRC asserts otherwise.

Privileged data

6.27 Legal privilege arises under common law and may only be overridden if this is expressly or necessarily implicitly set out in legislation. It protects a party's right to communicate in confidence with a legal adviser. The privilege belongs to the client and not to the member. If a document is privileged:

- The client cannot be required to make disclosure of that document to HMRC and a member should be careful to ensure that her reasons for advising a client nevertheless to make such a disclosure are recorded in writing.

- It must not be disclosed by any other party, including the member, without the clients express permission.

6.28 There are two types of legal privilege under common law, legal advice privilege covering documents passing between a client and her legal adviser prepared for the purposes of obtaining or giving legal advice and litigation privilege for data created for the dominant purpose of litigation. Litigation privilege may arise where litigation has not begun, but is merely contemplated and may apply to data prepared by non-lawyer advisers (including tax advisers) if brought into existence for the purposes of the litigation.

6.29 Communications from a tax adviser who is not a practising lawyer will not attract legal advice privilege but other similar protections exist under statute law, including:

- A privilege reporting exemption which applies to the reporting of money laundering in certain circumstances.

- A privilege under Schedule 36 whereby a tax adviser does not have to provide data that is her property and which constitute communications between the adviser and either her client or another tax adviser of the client. Information about such communications is similarly privileged. However, care should be taken as not all data may be privileged.

6.30 Whether data is or is not privileged and protected from the need to disclose is a complex issue, which will turn on the facts of the particular situation.

6.31 A member who receives a request for data, some of which she believes may be subject to privilege, should take independent legal advice on the position, unless expert in this area.

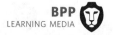

Bibliography

Association of Accounting Technicians (2016) *AAT Professional Diploma in Accounting Level 4 Qualification Specification.* [Online] Available from: www.aat.org.uk/prod/s3fs-public/assets/AAT_Professional_Diploma_in_Accounting_Level_4_Qualification_Specification.pdf [Accessed on 18 July 2016].

Association of Accounting Technicians (2016) *Personal Tax Professional conduct in relation to taxation reference material.* [Online] Available from: www.aat-interactive.org.uk/elearning/Sample_assessments_AQ2016/AQ2016_L4_PLTX_FA2016_reference_materials_PCRTT.pdf [Accessed on 18 July 2016].

Association of Accounting Technicians (2016) *Personal Tax Taxation tables for tasks 2–13.* [Online] Available from: www.aat-interactive.org.uk/elearning/Sample_assessments_AQ2016/AQ2016_L4_PLTX_FA2016_reference_materials_Tax_Tables.pdf [Accessed on 18 July 2016].

Association of Accounting Technicians (2016) *Sample Assessment AQ2016 PTAX FA15.* [Online] Available from: www.aat-interactive.org.uk/elearning/Sample_assessments_AQ2016/AQ2016_L4_PLTX_FA2016_Sample_1/index.html [Accessed on 18 July 2016].

Her Majesty's Revenue and Customs (2014) *Expenses & benefits: A tax guide.* [Online] Available from: www.gov.uk/government/uploads/system/uploads/attachment_data/file/314687/480-2014.pdf [Accessed on 16th August 2016].

Contains public sector information licensed under the Open Government Licence v3.0. www.nationalarchives.gov.uk/doc/open-government-licence/version/3/.

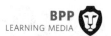

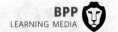

Index

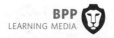

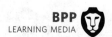

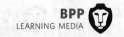

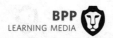

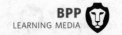

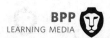

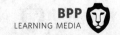

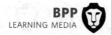

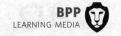

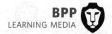

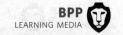

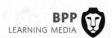

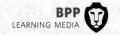

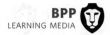

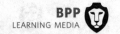

REVIEW FORM

How have you used this Course Book?
(Tick one box only)

☐ Self study

☐ On a course_____

☐ Other _____

Why did you decide to purchase this Course Book? *(Tick one box only)*

☐ Have used BPP materials in the past

☐ Recommendation by friend/colleague

☐ Recommendation by a college lecturer

☐ Saw advertising

☐ Other _____

During the past six months do you recall seeing/receiving either of the following?
(Tick as many boxes as are relevant)

☐ Our advertisement in Accounting Technician

☐ Our Publishing Catalogue

Which (if any) aspects of our advertising do you think are useful?
(Tick as many boxes as are relevant)

☐ Prices and publication dates of new editions

☐ Information on Course Book content

☐ Details of our free online offering

☐ None of the above

Your ratings, comments and suggestions would be appreciated on the following areas of this Course Book.

	Very useful	Useful	Not useful
Chapter overviews	☐	☐	☐
Introductory section	☐	☐	☐
Quality of explanations	☐	☐	☐
Illustrations	☐	☐	☐
Chapter activities	☐	☐	☐
Test your learning	☐	☐	☐
Keywords	☐	☐	☐

	Excellent	Good	Adequate	Poor
Overall opinion of this Course Book	☐	☐	☐	☐

Do you intend to continue using BPP Products? ☐ Yes ☐ No

Please note any further comments and suggestions/errors on the reverse of this page and return it to: Nisar Ahmed, AAT Head of Programme, BPP Learning Media Ltd, FREEPOST, London, W12 8AA.

Alternatively, the Head of Programme of this edition can be emailed at: nisarahmed@bpp.com.

REVIEW FORM (continued)

TELL US WHAT YOU THINK

Please note any further comments and suggestions/errors below